OXFORD MEDICAL PUBLICATIONS

Clinical Judgement

Clinical Judgement
Evidence in Practice

R. S. DOWNIE MA BPHIL FRSE FRSA
Professor of Moral Philosophy
University of Glasgow
Visiting Professor
Centre for Arts and Humanities in Health and Medicine
University of Durham

JANE MACNAUGHTON MA MB CHB MRCGP DRCOG PHD
Director
Centre for Arts and Humanities in Health and Medicine
University of Durham

and

FIONA RANDALL MB BS FRCP
Consultant in Palliative Medicine
Bournemouth and Christchurch Hospital Trust

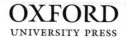

OXFORD
UNIVERSITY PRESS

OXFORD

UNIVERSITY PRESS

Great Clarendon Street, Oxford OX2 6DP

Oxford University Press is a department of the University of Oxford.
It furthers the University's objectives of excellence in research, scholarship,
and education by publishing worldwide in

Oxford New York
Athens Auckland Bangkok Bogotá Buenos Aires Calcutta
Cape Town Chennai Dar es Salaam Delhi Florence Hong Kong Istanbul
Karachi Kuala Lumpur Madrid Melbourne Mexico City Mumbai
Nairobi Paris São Paulo Singapore Taipei Tokyo Toronto Warsaw
and associated companies in Berlin Ibadan

Oxford is a registered trade mark of Oxford University Press
in the UK and in certain other countries

Published in the United States
by Oxford University Press, Inc., New York

A catalogue record for this title
is available from the British Library

Library of Congress Cataloging in Publication Data
Downie, R. S. (Robert Silcock)
Clinical judgement : evidence in practice / R.S. Downie, Jane Macnaughton,
and Fiona Randall.
(Oxford medical publications)
Includes bibliographical references and index.
1. Evidence-based medicine. 2. Clinical medicine–Decision making.
I. Macnaughton, Jane. II. Randall, Fiona. III. Title. IV. Series.
[DNLM: 1. Decision Making. 2. Judgment. 3. Evidence-Based Medicine. W 61
D751ca 2000]
RA425.D69 2000   616′.001–dc21   99-059423

ISBN 0 19 263216 7 (Pbk)

Typset by Downdell, Oxford
Printed in Great Britain
on acid-free paper by
Biddles Ltd,
Guildford & King's Lynn

Contents

Acknowledgements

We should like to acknowledge the help of several friends in the writing of this book. In particular, we should like to thank Dr Fiona Randall for providing a chapter on resource management or rationing. Fiona also commented on other aspects of the book and this provided us with the perspective of a hospital consultant on various issues. Some of our ideas are the outcome of previous collaborative projects: in particular with Professor Sir Kenneth Calman, Professor Frank Sullivan, Dr Bruce Charlton, Dr Blair Smith, and others. Their contributions are, of course, included in the references, but a reference does not always do justice to the help received. Finally, we would like to thank Frances Daw for her invaluable help with word processing.

Preface

There is a widespread view in medicine, and amongst the general public, that modern medicine is primarily a scientific enterprise and that the decisions of clinicians are determined by a secure foundation of evidence-based science. In terms of this view, the need for clinical judgement is minimal. The aims of this book are to make a case for the centrality and irreplaceabilty of clinical judgement, to identify the elements of good clinical judgement, and to suggest how these might be developed. Our aims might be stated in another way. There is an old adage that medicine is both a science and an art. We try to give a detailed explanation of what that means, and to show how the 'evidence-based medicine' movement can be integrated with the 'arts or humanities in medical education' movement. This integration provides the basis for the sound clinical judgements which are evidence in practice.

We shall begin by examining the scientific evidence-base of medicine. It will emerge that there are three aspects to medical science: first, systematic knowledge of the systems of the body and their pathology; second, descriptive studies including qualitative research; and third, randomized, controlled trials. Of the three, only the first is at the centre of science, but since the branches of science comprise a large family, randomized, controlled trials and qualitative research can be seen as members of the extended family. The nature of the evidence deriving from these more remote cousins of the science family will be of a different logical nature from that deriving from the nuclear family. In particular, we shall show that the attempt to quantify the evidence of qualitative research fails, and that the interpretation of that evidence requires a kind of judgement more akin to that of a literary critic than that of a core scientist. But the evidence suggested by any member of the science family, even of the nuclear family, can be shown not to be objectively 'out there' but to be a product of humane judgement, in the sense that interpretation and insight are required. The judgement here is the scientific or the technical component of clinical judgement.

We go on to ask how this scientific evidence-base is assimilated into clinical practice. It emerges that there must be a number of important modifications. First, evidence must be individualized to the specific patient. In discussing this we bring out that obsession with scientific paradigms in medicine can blind us to the existence of other helpful paradigms. One of these is that of the detective. The clinician uses evidence in the same way as a detective uses evidence in his investigation of a particular case. This sort of investigation into the particularities of a case is not any kind of science, although the clinician, like the detective, will use science. Second, doctors (like detectives) draw on wider sources of information than just the scientific evidence-base when they are treating patients. For example, patients' anecdotes and stories about themselves and the origins of their complaints are an important source of information in constant use. Third, all the information in use by doctors is interpreted by them in the light of their knowledge of, and insights into, the individual patient, and there is also an ethical dimension in that the patient's views must be sought on treatment decisions in the form of consent.

In adapting the scientific evidence-base to the clinical situation, and employing particularized evidence and other sources of information about the patient, it is clear that the doctor requires judgement of a technical sort. But, in addition to technical judgement, the good doctor must exercise what we call a 'humane judgement'. The elements of this derive here, as they did in the matter of scientific judgement, partly from the doctor's capacity for interpretation and insight. But humane judgement requires the additional factors of ethical sensitivity and a broad educational perspective. We analyse these elements of humane judgement. Clinical judgement is an amalgam of scientific and humane judgements, and that amalgam is evidence in practice.

It must be remembered that there is a domain in medicine other than the clinical, namely the public. The scientific evidence-base of public health medicine is epidemiology, which is often seen as the paradigm of objectivity. But judgement is also required in deciding what to do, if anything, about the figures suggested by epidemiological studies, and in deciding what figures should be collected in the first place. Epidemiology, therefore, is not immune to judgement.

The same is true of resource management or (crudely) health-care rationing. We have asked a hospital consultant, Dr Fiona Randall, to discuss this. She argues that there is overwhelming evidence for the need for rationing, a need based partly on financial considerations and partly on considerations of justice. But the implementation of rationing policies is very much a matter for the scientific and humane judgements of the clinician.

Can clinical judgement be taught? The scientific component can be taught (although the best way of doing so is still contro-versial) but it is less clear whether, and if so how, the components of humane judgement can be taught. Emphasis in medical education has concentrated on encouraging ethical awareness, but it is equally important that medical education, both under-graduate and postgraduate, should enable doctors to develop a broad perspective. Here the humanities have an important role to play, and this has recently been encouraged by the GMC and other bodies. This broad perspective is necessary if medical training is to become medical education.

The diagrammatic summary (see Figure 1 on the following page) illustrates the main lines of our argument. But it must be emphasized that the distinctions drawn between the element of the scientific and the element of the humane (and the sub-divisions within these boxes) are there for clarity of exposition. When evidence is in practice—or at least in best practice—clinical judgement operates as a unity.

Robin Downie
Jane Macnaughton

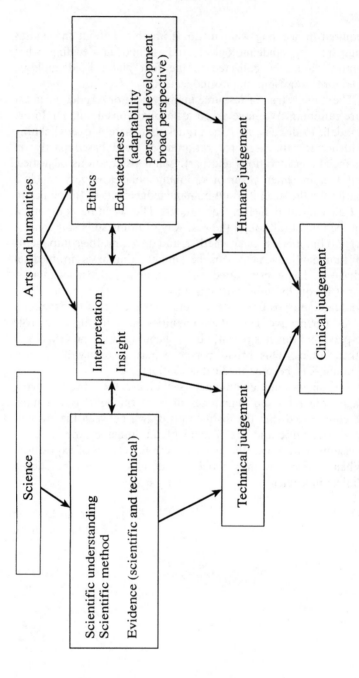

Figure 1 Clinical judgement: a diagrammatic summary.

1 Judgement and science

1.1 Introduction

Any account of what makes a good doctor must have something to say on scientific medicine. The good doctor, whatever else he may be, must at least be some sort of scientist. Now, whereas it is impossible to dissent from this view, it is a much more complex view than might seem to be the case. There are two complexities. First, the assimilation of science by medicine is relevant in different ways to medicine; the impact of science in medical research is different from its impact on clinical practice. In this chapter, we are concerned with science and medical research, and in the next chapter, with science and clinical practice. Second, different sorts of activities count in medical opinion as scientific. There are three activities regarded by doctors as comprising modern medical research:

(1) the search for systematic understanding of the body in its normal workings and in its pathology;

(2) observational studies, which may be divided into two subgroups:
  (a) quantitative studies, which include simple descriptive studies and also more complicated cohort and case-control studies of patient populations;
  (b) qualitative studies of the behaviour of patients, doctors, and their interactions;

(3) experimental studies, such as randomized trials, which involve an intervention.

It will emerge that judgement is integral to all three activities. Results are not objectively determined by science but to a greater or lesser extent require the interpretation and judgement of the researcher.

In order to discuss what is 'scientific' about activities (1)–(3), we will describe what is meant by 'science' in its general sense (Sections 1.2–1.6). We will then return to a discussion of the medical applications of science to the biological and pathological understanding of the body (Section 1.7.1), to the empirical observation of patient and doctor interactions (Section 1.7.2), and to the design, implementation, and dissemination of the results of scientific trials in medicine (Section 1.7.3). Having examined medicine with this scientific spotlight, we will conclude this chapter by offering an answer to the question, 'Is medicine scientific?' (Section 1.8). The answer will be that it is, but not to the extent that the need for judgement is eliminated.

1.2 The nature of science: method

The question, 'What is science?' is a difficult one to answer. It was not always so, however, because science at root means simply 'knowledge' from the Latin *scientia*. The problem we are addressing arises only from the beginning of the eighteenth century when there was an attempt to distinguish what we now mean by science from the rest of knowledge.

What emerges from an examination of the debate on the nature of science from the eighteenth to the twentieth centuries is that there is no one account that covers all the activities, aims, or methods that have been regarded as 'science'; rather, there is a range of such activities that have a legitimate claim to be called scientific. The implication of this position is that, rather than seek necessary and sufficient conditions, we shall do better to look for a range of 'family resemblances' or overlapping sets of characteristics that will link together to build up the concept of science. This method will be particularly useful in the context of the discussion of the scientific nature of medicine, as we will be able to refer to various sorts of scientific activity. This variety of activities will help illustrate the different ways in which medicine might be thought to be scientific. The variety emerges when we try to characterize science in terms of a method (Section 1.2), a kind of evidence (Section 1.3), an aim (Section 1.4), and an outlook (Section 1.5).

Many philosophers who wish to characterize the activities of science in terms of a method, begin by examining the features that emerged when science began to take its contemporary shape during the seventeenth and eighteenth centuries. This is not an unreasonable procedure because it is easier to detect the conceptual structure of science at this time than it is later, when the content of science had become technically much more complex and the separate sciences had adopted identities of their own. If we are to distinguish the wood from the trees, it is preferable to look at this early period. Yet there is one common failing in the philosophers who take this approach: it is that they are drawn in to the huge gravitational field of major scientists such as Galileo and Newton, and they define the characteristics of scientific method as a whole in terms of the characteristics of natural philosophy and its essential quantification. This, as we shall see (Section 1.7.3), has had a disastrous effect on some aspects of medical research. We shall try not to ignore the major contributions of Galileo and Newton, but shall also bear in mind those of biologists and natural historians.

1.2.1 Salient features of scientific method

There are a number of points to be made here. First, most scientific enquiries start with an *observation*, which—because science seeks to explain things about the world—is turned by the scientist in to a question. For example, the scientist might observe that when an object is dropped into a pool of water, concentric waves spread out from that point in ever-increasing circles until they decay. This observation then becomes a puzzle that must be solved. The second step in the process is to suggest an explanation as to why this might happen, i.e. to set up an hypothesis. In this case, the hypothesis might be that, in the process of dropping the stone into the pool, some energy is transferred to the water, which becomes wave energy that slowly decays the further it gets from the source of the energy.

Having set up the hypothesis, or possible explanation for the observation, the scientist in the third step has to test it by experiment to see if it is correct, or at least probable. His experimentation may confirm or deny his hypothesis. If the hypothesis is proved false, he will have to start again at step two with a new hypothesis and then test this one for its veracity.

The important point about this third step is that the experimentation is designed to prove that the explanation or hypothesis applies to *all* instances when the same circumstances exist. In other words, if, every time a stone was thrown into the water, the scientist was able to test his hypothesis about the outcome, he would come up with the same explanation time after time. So the fourth characteristic point about scientific method is that it produces conclusions that are generalizable and apply in all other similar circumstances. A discipline like history does not aim to produce conclusions that are applicable to all similar situations. The point about history is that each event must be studied on its own terms and in its own context. We may find that there are similarities in the circumstances that preceded the French and Russian revolutions, but we certainly cannot say that they were the same circumstances or that the explanation for both is the same.

At least some of the generalizations produced by science are called 'laws'. There are many types of scientific law. Perhaps the least complex of these scientific generalizations is at the level of what we might call 'natural history'—the observation that types of attribute tend to go together. For example, a doctor may observe that certain types of symptoms tend to go together, or that a certain type of treatment tends to be effective with certain types of disorder, or certain types of patient. No underlying causal explanation is offered. This sort of generalization is often dismissed as 'anecdotal' by the scientifically-minded, but it is precisely this sort of observation that is the starting point of medical science. It is a matter of no importance whether we regard such observations as 'scientific' or just as remote cousins of the science family.

We are moving more centrally into science when we reach observations dealing with uniformities of change or development. Laws of this kind are common in medicine. They might state, say, the stages in the development of an embryo or the course of a disease. For example, it is a law of the development of an embryo that the formation of the lungs never precedes the formation of the circulatory system.

Another type of law deals with numerical constants in nature. Into this group fall laws concerned with the melting points of chemical substances or the propagation of sound or light.

Yet another type of law deals with functional relationships between measurable quantities, such as the law that for any gas $PV = kT$ (where P stands for pressure, V for volume, T for absolute temperature, while k is a constant depending only on the units of measurement chosen). The functional relationship need not be simple but may be of any type recognized in mathematics, provided only that for each value of a certain variable or variables there should be only one value of another variable.

Quantitative laws of the last two types have been formulated only in the more recent stages of scientific development, and sometimes they can be regarded as refinements of previously known qualitative laws. For example, it was known in pre-historic times that iron melted at great heat, and a quantitative law expressing, on a scale of temperature, precisely at what point iron melts, can be regarded as a more precise formulation of this early perception. Again, it was known from early times that a projectile followed a curved path but Galileo was able to show that the path is a semi-parabola. More recently, some quantitative laws have been expressed statistically. Laws of this kind are to be found in physics, in biology, and, especially, in the social sciences. We shall find later that the results of randomized control trials are often expressed in statistical terms.

The importance of quantitative precision in science is so great that some scientists argue that no law is properly scientific unless it is purely quantitative. The arguments behind this view are: that true science must be precise and only the quantitative is precise; and that true science must be beyond the subjective, the realm of personal opinions, interpretations, and anecdotes, and only the quantitative takes us beyond this realm. These arguments are not convincing. First, laws such as the developmental ones earlier mentioned do not seem to be open to quantitative formulation, yet they are precise. Second, some laws, such as the statistical ones already mentioned, are quantitative but cannot be absolutely precise since they express only relative frequencies. Third, even the quantitative can be open to different interpretations, as is notorious in the case of statistical findings. It is naive to think that only the qualitative is controversial. We shall argue later (Section 1.7.3) that the desire to use numbers inappropriately can lead to serious distortion of qualitative research.

To sum up this discussion of generalizations in science, we can say that it is an essential feature of a scientific discipline that it attempts to provide generalizations, some of which can be called 'laws'. It emerged that at least five types of these law-like generalizations are used in science: the correlations noted in natural history or clinical observation; developmental laws; the establishment of numerical constants; laws of functional dependence; and statistical laws. Some of these generalizations or laws can legitimately be quantitative, but this is not essential to laws, far less to an activity's being called 'scientific'. It will be a constant theme in this book that the misplaced attempt to use numbers has led to distorted results in some medical research, especially qualitative research. What laws and generalization do, whether quantitative or not, is to contribute to the systematic understanding of natural processes, including disease processes.

Returning now to our discussion of the methods of scientific research, we have seen so far that it involves observation, the setting up of explanatory (generally causal) hypotheses, the testing of these by further observation, experiment or interventions, and the generalization of results into law-like form. We can now proceed to a fifth point about scientific research, which it is important to stress. The generalizations achieved by science depend on what we might call 'reductivism'. In order to generalize, the scientist or medical researcher must abstract from the bewildering complexity of nature one or a small set of features, which are the object of the generalization. What is generalized in a law is one or a small number of the same features. For example, when Newton tells us that a body will remain in a state of rest or of uniform motion in a straight line unless compelled to alter that state, he is abstracting rest and motion from the many features, such as air resistance, which an actual body might encounter, and he is dealing with one feature only of the body. It is not relevant that the body might be a

brightly coloured beach ball. Similarly, when a medical researcher is concerned with the statistical results of a randomized
controlled trial (RCT), he abstracts from the fact that in actual
life someone might do better on the pills because he knows that
his neighbour has used them and felt better, or because he trusts
his doctor. The researcher must ignore such contingencies, just as
Newton abstracts from the complexity of actual situations. But
in the real world, doctors use the treatments in the complexity of
actual clinical encounters. Hence, the evidence-based treatments
may do better or worse than the trial suggests because they
cannot but be reductivist, whereas clinical situations are holistic,
and constantly require the interpretation, insight and judgement
of the clinician.

In summary, then, scientific method usually takes the form of:

(1) observation;

(2) hypothesis formation;

(3) experimentation, which if it confirms or, at least, renders
possible the hypothesis, leads to:

(4) generalization, which requires:

(5) reductivism.

This outline describes the whole scientific process, but often
scientific 'method' is taken to mean the experimental methods
used by scientists. We will say more about this in Section 1.3.2
but will note here that most people regard the methods of science
as primarily quantitative. This is the main reason why the col-
loquial sense of science has the meanings it now has of 'precision'
and 'reliability'. However, qualitative research methods are now
being used in some scientific disciplines in order to measure
things that are not amenable to numerical measurement. This
movement has a bearing now on research work in medicine and
we will assess in a later section (1.7.3) the extent to which this
might be regarded as scientific or not.

Note also that in RCTs, the hypothesis may be only that, what
has been observed to be successful in a few clinical situations,
may be successful in a majority of situations. In other words, the
hypothesis is non-causal. An hypothesis of this kind is clearly
less satisfactory as science than a causal hypothesis. Hence,

RCTs, far from being a 'gold standard' of science, can never be part of the nuclear family of science.

We have so far been concerned with scientific method but should note here for completeness that, in addition to using the method, a scientist must be impartial, rigorous, and detached. These characteristics belong, of course, to the practitioners of other disciplines, such as that of the historian, but they are certainly essential to the scientist, and as such we shall discuss them when we discuss the scientific outlook (Section 1.5), but note that the impartiality, rigour, and detachment of researchers are good reasons for trusting their judgements.

1.3   Evidence

A central concept of scientific method is 'evidence'. The reason why some analysis of the concept of evidence is necessary here is that the scientific pretensions of medicine are currently expressed via the concept of evidence. 'Evidence-based medicine' has become a catch-phrase, which cannot be questioned in medical circles. But what is 'evidence' and what is its place in science?

Our method of analysis will be to investigate the logical process that converts inconsequential facts into 'evidence', and in so doing we shall discuss the proper use of the different strands of evidence that are available to the practising physician. In order to illuminate the nature of evidence, as it is seen in medicine, we shall draw parallels with 'evidence' as understood in science and in detective work.

From one point of view, evidence is really just information, but it is a certain kind of information in that it relates to a *specific* medical, scientific, or forensic conclusion. We do not just say, 'This is evidence', we say, 'This is evidence *for* something or *that* something is the case'. Information and data can be about something but they do not suggest that we must draw any con-clusions from them. A couple of examples might help to outline the process by which data becomes evidence.

Henry's friend comes round to visit him one evening and gets no answer when he rings the bell. The friend looks for Henry's car and finds that it is gone. Being persistent, he checks round at

Henry's back door and finds it locked and that the kitchen lights are out, and the house is silent. The friend assesses all this data in the context of his attempted visit and concludes that Henry is out. The facts of the unanswered bell, the absent car, and the darkened house, therefore, become evidence that Henry is away from home.

To take a legal example, in the case against McTavish, who is alleged to have held up and robbed a bank, the prosecuting lawyer says, 'The facts in the case are these: McTavish bought a gun; he was seen in the region of the bank at the time of the armed robbery; he was later found in possession of a large sum of money'. These facts become evidence when the lawyer suggests that the jury must conclude that it was McTavish who held up the bank.

What, then, are the important aspects of the handling of the facts in these two cases which turn them into evidence? First, the facts have to be relevant to the case and they must be relevant in a particular way, i.e. in that they are facts that contribute to a specific hypothesis relating to the case. The three facts in the first case (the unanswered bell, the absent car, and the darkened house) are all relevant to the claim that Henry is not at home and they suggest that conclusion. Second, there must be some assessment of the extent to which these facts suggest this conclusion. We will refer to this aspect of evidence as its 'weight'. For example, facts may be relevant to a case but we have to know *how* relevant they are in order to assess whether these facts are more or less likely to support the hypothesis we have formed. If we look again at the second example, the fact that McTavish was seen in the region of the bank at the time it was robbed might be said to be relevant to the hypothesis that it was he who robbed the bank, but there were also many other people walking up and down outside the bank at that time. However, as we are able to bring forward other bits of information that are relevant to our hypothesis—McTavish had bought a gun and he was found in possession of a large sum of money—the importance or weight of this first piece of evidence increases.

The third and final point about the handling of facts as evidence is that they must be submitted to the judgement of an assessor.[1] This seems an obvious point in view of the above

discussion because it is necessary to submit facts to the judgement of someone who will carry out the process of assessing their
relevance as evidence, weighing their importance, and drawing
conclusions from them. This point needs to be stressed, however,
as it is an important point of distinction between facts and evidence. Facts or data can be accepted without recourse to judgement but facts as evidence necessarily involve judgement. The
concept of evidence is, therefore, parasitic upon the concept of
judgement. Now the concept of judgement is normative in the
sense that it is prioritizing certain facts as the important ones, or
it is claiming that certain facts amount to good evidence or put a
conclusion beyond reasonable doubt. We can, therefore, say that
the concept of evidence (which relies upon judgement) must also
be normative. In other words, the conclusion that some fact or
piece of data constitutes 'evidence' for something is not arrived
at through an entirely objective process, it depends on some
individual or group evaluation.

From this analysis we might say that 'evidence' is information
relating to a subject or case, which is relevant to a particular
argument and which gives weight to a certain conclusion about
the subject. The existence of facts as 'evidence' is, therefore,
irresistibly related to the concept of 'judgement' as someone has
to determine whether the facts are relevant and whether, and to
what extent, the facts support a certain conclusion. A collection
of data cannot, therefore, be called evidence until the context in
which it is to be used is clear and some process of reasoning has
been exerted to determine its usefulness in that context. Let us
now look at this process in more detail.

1.3.1 Relevance

The first thing to establish about information that might be used
as evidence is its relevance. It is important to be clear exactly
what we mean by 'relevance' in this context, as the concept can
have two meanings. The first is that the information has a
general association with the subject matter in that it is in some
non-specific way related to it. An example might be the
suggestion that blood-cholesterol levels are associated with the
development of heart disease in some way. The second meaning

is that the information is relevant only in the context of a specific hypothesis relating to the subject. In this case, the example would be that blood-cholesterol levels are related to heart disease in that a high level is associated with an increased likelihood of heart disease. The first meaning of relevance would not fit in with the conditions we have already established for data to be regarded as evidence. Data can also be *about* a subject, but evidence must relate to some hypothesis about the subject.

This second, more precise, meaning has implications for the way in which data is collected to be used as evidence, particularly in the context of a scientific inquiry. If, as we have argued, data must be relevant to a specific hypothesis about a subject to be used as evidence, then the hypothesis must be formulated *before* the collection of the data. If it is not, then the enquirer has no idea whether the information he is collecting, or the context in which he is studying it, will be relevant to his study or not. The philosopher of science, Carl Hempel, summarizes this point :

An empirical finding is relevant for a hypothesis if and only if it constitutes either favourable or unfavourable evidence for it; in other words if it either confirms or disconfirms the hypothesis.[2]

The implication of this conclusion is that scientific inquiry is not just about gathering together all the information we have about a subject and seeing where it takes us. We have to construct an hypothesis and use only that information which is relevant to the hypothesis and, as Hempel has said, the information is still evidence even if it disconfirms the hypothesis. This way of looking at evidence is particularly relevant to a scientific inquiry and we might, therefore, call it the 'science model' of evidence.

It is, however, possible to argue for the first meaning of relevance in other contexts where evidence is used. The work of the detective is one such context. In Arthur Conan Doyle's *A Study in Scarlet*, Dr Watson upbraids Sherlock Holmes for not paying enough attention to the case they have just set out to investigate:

'You don't seem to give much thought to the matter in hand,' I said at last, interrupting Holmes's musical disquisition.

'No data yet,' he answered. 'It is a capital mistake to theorize before you have all the evidence. It biases the judgement.'[3]

The role of the detective, as described here by Holmes, is to amass all the material relating to a case and then formulate some hypothesis as to its solution. Once there is sufficient evidence to form the hypothesis that Jones has committed, the crime then the detective can set about trying to prove a case against Jones. This model of evidence contrasts with the science model, described above, in that the hypothesis is derived from a consideration of the evidence available.

In summary, we now have two models of 'relevant' evidence. One, which we have called the 'science model', says that data are relevant as evidence for a hypothesis only if they contribute to a specific argument for or against that hypothesis. The second, which we might call the 'detective model', says that all data are relevant if they have some bearing on a case and can contribute to the formation of a hypothesis relating to that case. We will come back to these ideas later when considering the idea of judgement.

1.3.2 Weight

Moving from the two models of 'relevance', we can now consider the second factor about the concept of evidence: this is the 'weight' to be given to information considered as evidence. Having established that a hypothesis 'H' may be corroborated by a body of evidence 'E' (which is what we would attempt to do by establishing relevance), we then need to move on to establish the *extent* to which E confirms H. This will enable us to decide whether hypothesis H is a more plausible explanation of events or phenomena than another hypothesis, H1. Hempel breaks the problem of defining weight into two parts:

(1) to lay down criteria defining a metrical concept 'degree of confirmation of H with respect to E', whose values are real numbers; or failing this,

(2) to lay down criteria defining two relational concepts, 'more highly confirmed than' and 'equally well confirmed as', which make possible a non-metrical comparison of hypotheses.[4]

In the medical context, Hempel's first part might refer to any standard, randomized, controlled trial, where the outcomes can be measured numerically. Statistical calculations can be made on the probabilities of these outcomes coming about because of the drug being used in the trial (main hypothesis) or because of chance (alternative hypothesis). The statistical calculations used to represent such probabilities are p values and are appropriate for quantitative studies. Hempel's second part would be appropriate to qualitative studies, where the concern of the researcher is with concepts such as patient satisfaction or students' anxiety. A non-metrical comparative approach is appropriate for such studies as the concepts they deal with cannot be given numerical values in a meaningful way (see Section 1.7.3) and another method of expressing the degree of weight to be given to the evidence is required.

There is, therefore, no single correct approach to assessing the weight to be given to evidence in medicine. At times it is appropriate to apply numerical calculations to the solution and at other times the best that can be said is 'more probable' or 'less probable'.

1.3.3 Judgement

So far we have looked at the process by which a body of information or data becomes evidence when its relevance and weight with respect to a certain hypothesis are established. Now we come to look at the way in which this relevance is established and importance weighed, i.e. through the personal judgement of the investigator:

The investigator's task is to assemble the relevant evidence and then to judge whether the assay means A or B: true or false, innocent or guilty, well or ill. The historian, the judge, the physician follow methodological procedures that hinge upon a common characteristic: their personal judgement must play the decisive role in assembling the evidence, drawing the inference, and formulating the conclusion in each case they consider.[5]

In this passage, Lerner emphasizes the importance of personal judgement at all stages of the process by which data becomes

evidence. The importance of, and elements in, personal judgement will be discussed again in Sections 2.6, 3.6 and in Chapter 7.
We stress the importance of these factors because they are the
key to our analysis of good clinical judgement.

Let us, therefore, look at the role of judgement in relation to
the two models of evidence that we considered earlier, when
considering relevance. The scientist relies on the prior creation of
an hypothesis, which could be tested experimentally to establish findings that should be true in all similar circumstances.
The time for personal judgement in this model is at the
formulation of the hypothesis, which precedes data collection.
The hypothesis itself might come about as a result of a flash of
insight[6] (see Section 3.6.2) or from a period of contemplation,
but it requires the exercise of the investigator's judgement to
assess whether it is worth experimental testing and in what way.
This approach can be described as 'hypothetico-deductive'
reasoning. The detective model relies on the amassing of all
relevant information in a case for consideration by the
investigator who would then construct an argument relating
to the case. The hypothesis formation follows a consideration
of the relevant data and might be described as inductive
reasoning.

The two models differ, therefore, in the kind of thinking that
results from their approach to the concept of relevance. If we
consider also the question of the aim of science, as distinct from
that of detective work, we find a further fundamental distinction:
the scientist aims at establishing truths about the world that will
hold in all similar circumstances; the detective looks only to
discover the truth in the particular case he is considering. Those
specific truths will have no universal applications, though the
experience of studying the particular case may be of use to the
detective in future cases. The distinction between the scientist's
and the detective's approach to, and inferences from, evidence
will come up again in Section 2.4. But it is clear that both rely on
personal judgement; judgement cannot be eliminated by evidence
because the very concept depends on the prior exercise of
judgement. This is scientific or technical or forensic judgement
and, as we shall see, it is one of the two components of good
clinical judgement.

1.4 Scientific aims

1.4.1 Understanding

We have so far tried to characterize science in terms of methods and procedures, including the use of evidence. But another way of identifying science is in terms of its aims. We wish to maintain that the primary aim of scientists is to reach a particular kind of understanding of nature, including human nature and society. This aim is intrinsic to, or internal to, scientific activity as such, although of course some scientists may wish to apply their understanding to goals external to science, such as finding cures or building bridges. The understanding of the scientist derives from systematic knowledge, from knowledge of the 'connecting principles' of nature (see Section 1.6).

By saying that scientific knowledge is systematic, we mean that each bit of knowledge is known and understood in relation to other bits of knowledge, and is dependent on other knowledge and understanding. The systematic understanding of the natural and biological sciences is typically (although not necessarily) causal. If we compare science with natural history, this may become clearer. We could suggest that the aims of natural history and science are the same: to discover the truth about the world. The naturalist might make the observation that insectivorous plants are to be found commonly in boggy ground. This observation is sufficient for the naturalist, whose role is to describe what it is that he sees. The scientist (botanist in this context), however, would go further and wish to explain this observation. He might suggest from other knowledge that, as boggy ground is nitrogen-poor, the plants that inhabit it need to get their nitrogen from somewhere else so they devour insects. The botanist could go on to test this theory for its validity. The natural historian's observation does not need to be part of other knowledge; it can stand on its own. The scientist, however, is interested in building the knowledge of his subject into a systematic whole, where each aspect makes sense in the context of the rest and must be understood in the light of the rest. Typically, as in the botanical example, the systematic understanding is causal.

1.4.2 Control

The origins of the view that the aim of science is to control nature for human betterment are to be found in the works of Francis Bacon (1561–1626). Bacon was not himself much of a scientist, but rather a prophet, or philosopher of science, and as such his writings were influential. His writings about science had three overlapping themes. First, he is caustic in his criticism of existing and preceding science:

For the wit and mind of man, if it work upon matter, which is the contemplation of the creatures of God, worketh according to the stuff and is limited thereby; but if it work upon itself, as the spider worketh his web, then it is endless, and brings forth indeed cobwebs of learning, admirable for the fineness of thread and work, but of no substance or profit.[7]

Second, he holds that science can proceed only by observation and experiment:

Man is the helper and interpreter of nature. He can only act and understand in so far as he has observed nature's order practically or theoretically. Outside this he has no knowledge or power.[8]

Third, and most relevantly for present purposes, he asserts the view that the justification for scientific research is to improve life for mankind.

It is well to observe the force and effect and consequences of discoveries. These are to be seen nowhere more conspicuously than in those three which were unknown to the ancients, and of which the origin, though recent, is obscure: namely, printing, gunpowder, and the magnet... no empire, no sect, no star seems to have exerted greater influence on human affairs than these mechanical inventions.[9]

It should be noted that Bacon did not clearly distinguish between the last two, and writes:

Truth therefore and utility are here the very same thing: and works themselves are of greater value as pledges of truth, than as contributions to the comforts of life.[10]

This view, that the aim of science is to control nature for 'human welfare', had a large following in the eighteenth century, and many intellectual societies were established with that aim. For example, the Royal Society of Edinburgh was founded in 1783 with the aim of 'the advancement of useful knowledge'. It is very much the view of contemporary research funding bodies.

The two views, that the aim of science is to provide understanding of nature through systematic knowledge, and that the aim is to control nature for human betterment, are not necessarily incompatible. For if we understand the workings of the natural world we may be able to use that systematic knowledge to control nature. This would be called 'applied science'. But in practice there are likely to be important differences between proponents of the two views in what is regarded as satisfactory science.

This contrast in the aims of science will be important when we come to examine the nature of scientific medicine, but we wish here to insist that 'applied science' is parasitic on pure science. The physicist is fundamentally different in his aim from the jobbing electrician, although both are important. The point is that the goals of the electrician and engineer are external to science, and follow from social purposes, whereas those of the scientist proper are internal to science and follow from the human impulse to understand and find the 'connecting principles of nature' (Section 1.6). Moreover, and this will become more central in the next section, the view that the aim of science is simply to understand, is psychologically, if not logically, connected with the view that the true scientist is detached from vested interests. That is one reason why, as we shall go on to discuss, there is public opinion in favour of the scientific outlook.

1.5 The scientific outlook

We have so far tried to characterize science in terms of a method, an approach to evidence, and an aim. Can it be characterized in terms of an outlook or general view of the world? It is certainly widely believed that there is such a thing as a scientific worldview. But when we examine what that is we find that it seems to be some one or combination of the points we have already made: that a certain method is involved, that strict criteria of evidence are used, or that the scientist is detached or disinterested. There is, however, an ambiguity in the public consciousness as to whether this world view is entirely a good thing. Our main concern in this chapter is with the analysis of what science *is* but the question of the public perception of science and scientific method is sufficiently important to justify a slight digression. We shall, therefore, examine briefly the ambiguity in the public view of science.

Take first the strand in public consciousness that depicts science as benign. It is an accepted point of advertising jargon to suggest that science has been applied in the making of a new product and that science has been involved in proving its effectiveness. For example, claims such as 'This shampoo is scientifically proven to cure dandruff' are common in advertising. This suggestion is frequently accompanied on screen by images of people wearing white coats and handling test tubes. The appeal of the advert is not, however, to the public's understanding of the technical aspects of the chemistry of a product, but to a general sense that science brings with it safety, reliability, and a certain guarantee that the thing will work. 'Science' has come to carry this meaning in everyday use because it is seen by most people as being the preserve of clever experts whose ways are mysterious to most ordinary people. The outcome of their activities, therefore, is mysterious and unfathomable to the ordinary mortal. This sense of 'science' is not just found in the advertising world; it is part of our everyday language. We will often say things like: 'Let's just be scientific about this', meaning, 'Let's just try to sort this out in a methodical and organized way'. Usually the epithet 'scientific' also carries the sense of 'better', as in: 'I prefer to do it your way; it's more scientific'.

To describe something as 'scientific', therefore, in this sphere of everyday speech, is to suggest that it is of proven benefit, reliable or just that it is better than something else or than some other way of proceeding. It is important to acknowledge this view of science in the context of this discussion because it implies that science is held in high regard by the public and that scientists can speak with some authority in the public domain. Medicine is perceived as an activity that relies on science, and people's trust in their doctors is partly based on this perception. The 'view of the scientist' is frequently sought in discussion programmes on issues of importance to society, and it is done for many reasons, some of which are connected with the ways in which we have already characterized science: in terms of its method, its strict approach to evidence, and its detached aim of systematic under-standing. In the public perception these qualifications entitle scientists to be seen as 'experts' and, because of their allegedly detached expertise, they are often invited by governments and other bodies to give advice on matters about which they have no special knowledge; the 'method' is held to be universally applicable. It is not thought by the public that science removes the need for judgement, but rather the thought is that the judgements of scientists are likely to be more reliable.

There is something to be said for this public perception. Take, for example, the views of scientists on the ethical issues of the day. Certainly, scientists are no more entitled than the rest of us to comment on the principles of ethics, but in some contexts they may be better placed to comment on the application of these principles. For public policy, and many areas of ethical debate, nowadays require knowledge of a sort that only scientists have. This knowledge gives the scientist the ability to have a view on certain issues that are not accessible to most people. For instance, the issue of xenotransplantation involves the creation of genetically manipulated pigs, whose organs might be used for transplantation into humans. There are clearly technical and practical points that only scientists can discuss in relation to this new technique, but the view of the scientist also needs to be sought regarding the ethics of such a procedure. The ethics of the technique are intimately connected with practical and technical issues, such as the extent to which new viruses might be passed from the animal to the human recipients of organs and so into the human domain. Thus the scientist as expert cannot simply confine himself to providing information; he must be prepared to consider the effects of the new knowledge that he has brought to light.

The example of xenotransplantation enables us to introduce the side to our perception of science that is less trusting. The first aspect of this concerns the assumption that scientists are concerned with the detached understanding of the world. Science nowadays involves big money, which comes from governments, large foundations, and pharmaceutical companies. There is a widespread suspicion that scientists can be corrupted by money as much as the rest of us. For example, pharmaceutical companies are anxious to make a return on their large investments and they, therefore, may be over-zealous in putting on the market products that are inadequately tested. There have been tragic examples of this, such as the thalidomide cases. Medicine is indeed especially liable to this undesirable aspect of science because of the competition among scientists to be first in the market with profit-making pharmaceuticals. This is unfortunate to the extent that it undermines our belief in the objectivity of scientific judgement.

A second, and connected, undesirable aspect of the scientific outlook concerns the fear that the impulse to control nature (Section 1.4.2) may lead scientists to 'play God' and thus tamper with what they only imperfectly understand. For example, the scientists of the day assured us of the desirable consequences of developing a nuclear industry. They were totally wrong. Are their successors, therefore, to be believed in issues such as xenotransplantation, cloning, or genetic engineering? We shall not here take sides on such issues but note them as examples of doubts, which make the general public suspicious of 'the scientific outlook' and the judgements which may follow from it.

A third aspect of science that is not thought to be wholly benign, accepts the 'control' view of science and further suggests that scientific procedures, scientists themselves, and the scientific outlook, are cold, unimaginative, uncreative, and boring.

On the other hand, the focus more recently has been on the similarities rather than on the differences in the intellectual culture of the arts and the sciences. The 'humanities in medicine' movement in medical education (Section 6.9) is part of this cultural shift but it is to be found in other areas too. Historians of science now emphasize the role of imagination, metaphor, and analogy in scientific thinking. Creativity is seen as much a part of scientific discovery as of artistic endeavour, and sudden insights as important for scientific judgement as for art. It seems a recent idea, but like so many 'recent' ideas it can be found in the

Scottish Enlightenment, and it is in that context that we shall discuss it. It Let us examine further the place of the imagination in scientific thinking.

1.6 Science and the imagination: Adam Smith

The idea that scientific thinking involves the imagination can be found in the Scottish Enlightenment, specifically in an essay by Adam Smith on the 'History of astronomy'.[11] The clue to Smith's intentions in this early essay is provided by the fuller title of his essay, 'The principles which lead and direct philosophical inquiries illustrated by the history of astronomy'. The term 'philosophy' must, of course, be taken here in a wide sense to include the natural sciences, but the important point for present purposes is Smith's use of the phrase 'lead and direct' philosophical inquiries. He means that he is offering what we might now regard as an account of the psychology of scientific discovery—the motivation of the scientist. We have so far characterized science in terms of a set of procedures and in terms of its aims. We can now characterize it in terms of a particular sort of motivation, a curiosity that is analysed by Smith in a novel way. Smith's account enables us to make a bridge between the scientist and the artist via the work of imagination.

Smith identifies three, what he calls, 'sentiments', which he thinks explain the psychology of scientific discovery. They are: 'wonder', 'surprise', and 'admiration'. He explains their operations as follows:

What is new and singular, excites that sentiment which, in strict propriety, is called Wonder; what is unexpected, Surprise; and what is great or beautiful, Admiration'.[12]

He has much of interest to say about all three of these 'sentiments', which indeed overlap and support each other, but it is his discussion of wonder that contains points of interest on scientific discovery and explanation. For present purposes, his argument may be summarized as follows.

The mind takes pleasure in observing resemblances between objects and consequently in arranging these resembling ideas into classes, technically called 'genera' and 'species'. The greater our knowledge, the more divisions and subdivisions we ascribe to genera and species. When something new turns up, this generates wonder when we try to assign it to some familiar class. There is a second kind of wonder. The first kind is generated when we encounter unusual individual entities, and the second kind when we encounter uncommon successions or trains of entities. This second kind is also generated by interruptions of customary successions with which the imagination is familiar. This is where the imagination has a role, for it steps in to fill the gaps in these interruptions. The imagination is then enabled to 'flow smoothly' along apparently disjointed events. Philosophers (scientists) who have spent their lives studying connecting principles between objects will often be aware of intervals between objects, which less informal or more careless observers will think are strictly conjoined. Philosophy is, therefore, the 'science of the connecting principles of nature'.[13] Chaotic events or irregularities disturb the imagination.

Philosophy (science), therefore may be regarded as one of those arts which address themselves to the imagination ...[14]

We can take from Smith the point that science is one of the arts that address themselves to the imagination, and what pleases the imagination is systematic understanding.

1.7 Medicine and science

Granted that we have roughly characterized science from various standpoints, historical and logical, we can now turn to the question, How far is medicine scientific? Medicine, of course, has a clinical as well as a research side, and we shall discuss the clinical side to medicine in Chapter 2. But let us now consider how far medical *research* can be considered scientific. It will be recalled that we began this chapter by noting that there are three areas of medical research:

(1) the search for systematic understanding of the body in its normal workings and in its pathology;

(2) observational studies, both quantitative and qualitative;

(3) experimental studies, in particular, randomized trials to establish the best treatments.

Let us discuss them in order.

1.7.1 Basic biology and pathology

If we take (1), we have an easy answer: the search for systematic understanding of the normal and pathological workings of the body is, obviously, completely scientific. The doctors involved are straightforwardly doing science with all the means and methods of contemporary science. Thus, normal and pathological biochemistry, physiology, anatomy, and so on, provide the developing and systematic scientific knowledge base of medicine, using all the methods of scientific research with the aim of providing understanding and reliable judgements about the workings of the body and its pathology. When we move to (2) and (3), however, we encounter more difficulty in reaching an appropriate answer. Let us begin with (2), observational studies, and discuss the two subsets of this kind of study: quantitative studies, which include simple descriptive studies, and case-control and cohort studies; and qualitative research.

1.7.2 Observational studies using quantitative methods

Although RCTs and qualitative studies are becoming more frequent in the medical literature, observational studies are still in the majority. They are simpler to do, less costly than RCTs, and, as they do not involve an intervention—i.e. there is no experimentation on their human subjects—do not have ethical implications. Observational studies can be simple in design, like surveys which take a cross-sectional look at a specific population of patients at a particular time, or more complex, like cohort and case-control studies. Let us turn first to the simpler descriptive studies and examine their scientific credentials.

Simple descriptive studies are carried out to provide answers to questions like, 'How often does disease x occur in population y?', and 'How does the prevalence of disease x in population y

compare with 10 years ago?'. Such questions can be answered
by looking at data collected routinely, such as NHS hospital
discharge forms (SMR2 forms) or general practice disease
registers, and do not necessarily require to be collected in a
planned way.

One example might be a study on the changes in birthweights
in Scotland between 1980 and 1992.[15] The investigators looked
at discharge sheets for maternity admissions for 94% of live
births in Scotland between these two dates and found that mean
birthweight had increased over this period from 3326 g to 3382 g.
Having made this observation, the investigators then went on to
try to answer the question, 'Why are babies getting heavier?' by
looking at associations with maternal height, age, and parity,
and they claim to show that these variables had an 'effect' on
birthweight. It is at this point that the study parts company with
our characterization of science. Judgements about the conclusions to be drawn might vary.

Descriptive studies, such as the above example, can only go
as far as satisfy the first two credentials of scientific method,
i.e. observation and hypothesis formation. The study on birthweights made the observation that babies were getting bigger and
asked the question, 'Why?'. The suggestion was made that this
finding might have 'something to do' with increasing maternal
height and age but this can only be posed as a hypothesis, which
would require further investigation to prove. There may be any
number of other correlations that might be significant in relation
to birthweight but which could not be taken into account
because they do not happen to be recorded on the SMR2 form.
One example quoted by the researchers is maternal smoking,
information on which was not collected before 1992. It may be
that these correlations are *likely* but just by showing that the
birthweight of babies is increasing *at the same time* as maternal
height does not mean that a *causal* association is proved. It may
be that, if consumption of Irn Bru or other sugary drinks were
recorded on the SMR2 form, an association might be found
between this and birthweight, but it is difficult to see how this
could be causal.

This point becomes clearer when we look at another cross-
sectional study suggesting a less likely correlation between the

taking of antibiotics and risk of heart attack.[16] This study was a retrospective analysis of data from 350 general practices in the UK and it suggested that patients who had no other risk factors for heart attack were less likely to have one if they had received certain antibiotics. Most readers would need some persuading to believe that this was a true correlation, as the casual mechanism of the association is not as clear as that between maternal height and birthweight. The point is that such studies cannot progress beyond the steps of observation and hypothesis formation, and researchers must be careful to avoid claims that they can. It is up to the researcher to interpret the results and pass (sometimes controversial) judgements about them.

The study on heart-attack risk involved a control group and would be described as a case-control study, which involves comparing people who have a disease (cases) with those who do not (controls). Case-control studies and cohort studies represent the more sophisticated forms of observational research. Case-control studies are often retrospective, whereas cohort studies involve prospective follow-up of groups of patients to find out what happens to them. Cohort studies require that there is already some hypothesis formed about the disease process or risk factor under investigation, so that the study can be designed to look for these. This hypothesis might have come from pre-liminary investigation in the form of a descriptive study. For instance, if the birthweight study had revealed a possible link between Irn Bru consumption and birthweight, a cohort study might be set up to test out this hypothesis. A group of pregnant Irn Bru drinkers would be identified along with a similar control group of non-drinkers and both would be followed up, with careful recording of amount of Irn Bru drunk, to determine the eventual weight of the babies. The careful isolation and recording of the risk factor makes a causal association more likely, but still not proved. Once again, judgement is necessary to interpret the results.

One of the most famous cohort studies is that by Doll *et al.*, which looked at the development of cancer in British doctors who smoked.[17] This study made observations that could not have been made if the researchers had used a simple descriptive design. First, they were able to show that the development of

cancers, mainly of the lung, *followed* the exposure to the risk
factor, and second, that there was as association between the
number of cigarettes smoked and the risk of cancer; in other
words there was a *dose-response* effect.[18] These observations
clearly make the hypothesis under consideration—that smoking
causes lung cancer—much more probable but it still does not
prove it. This proof would require the further step of experimentation in the process of scientific investigation. In other
words, descriptive studies, even those that use numbers, are not
scientific in the full sense; they remain at the natural history end
of science. In Section 1.7.4, we will examine the 'experimental'
aspect of this sort of descriptive medical research, the
randomized, controlled trial, and discuss whether this kind of
medical research fulfils all the prerequisites for science. But we
must stress here that in this kind of research, interpretation of
the results and judgement about what may be concluded are
necessary.

1.7.3 Observational studies using qualitative methods

Research that attempts to find the meaning behind a patient's or
a doctor's action, or to interpret their actions, is referred to
as 'qualitative research'. In the field of research on sexually
transmitted diseases, for example, a simple descriptive study
would answer the question, 'What is the prevalence in young
women of infection with *Chlamydia trachomatis*?'; whereas
qualitative methods would be required to find out what these
women understood about this infection and whether having had
the infection changed their behaviour in any way. Such methods
might include semi-structured interviews with individual women
and focus-group discussions.

There are really two questions involved in considering the
scientific credentials of qualitative research. First, can qualitative
research meaningfully use measurements and scales in the
manner of quantitative research?[19] Second, supposing we cannot
meaningfully use scales and measurements, does it follow that
quantitative research is not scientific? It is important to stress
that there are two questions here, for there is a tendency among
medical researchers to assume that what cannot be quantified

cannot count as 'real' science. But, as we have already suggested (Section 1.2), an activity can be scientific without being quantitative. Let us therefore examine the first question.

Should researchers involved in qualitative research use numbers to present their findings? There is an increasing focus on qualitative research in medicine[20] and, whereas the results of such research used to appear only in sociological, educational, and anthropological journals,[21] medical journals are beginning to publish some examples.[22] The problem is that doctors have been brought up (in a research sense) on the methods of quantitative research and these methods are given higher value than those of qualitative research by those who hold the purse-strings of funding and promotion—the editorial boards of medical journals.[23] (So much for detached, scientific understanding!) There is, therefore, a tendency to force qualitative research into a quantitative mould. For example, we find qualities like 'patient-centredness' being given a score of 1.45[24] and doctor satisfaction measured as 8.95.[25] Are such measurements meaningful or helpful?[26] In answering this question we shall focus on the uses of numbers and the establishment of scales, look at the implications numbers and scales have for qualitative research, and finally, suggest a more satisfactory interpretation of the findings of qualitative research.

Numbers and scales

Measurement has been defined as the correlation with numbers of entities which are not numbers.[27]

The use of numbers and the mechanism of counting are essential first steps in understanding the nature of measurement.

We use numbers in three distinct ways.[28] First, as a method of identification or labelling, as in the numbering of football players on a field or in labelling diagrams. In this case, the numbers have no relationship with each other and they are assigned in a totally arbitrary fashion.

Second, numbers are used to indicate the position of something in a series. Examples here might be the numbering of theatre seats or house numbers. The numbers indicate the relationship of one seat or house to the other, and enable people to find them easily. A more complex example of the same use of numbers is that of the relative hardness of wood, glass, and diamond. Diamond can cut glass but glass cannot cut diamond; glass can cut wood but wood cannot cut glass. We can, therefore, arrange these three objects in a series of increasing hardness, with wood at the bottom and diamond at the top. If we give wood the number 1, glass 2, and diamond 3, this tells us that wood is softer than glass, which is in turn softer than diamond. This kind of arrangement in a series is appropriate for non-additive qualities like hardness and also applies to the kinds of things that qualitative research deals with, such as patient satisfaction and quality of life. But the arrangement has a limitation: it does not tell us that diamond is three times as hard as wood because our series gives no indication of how much harder these objects are than each other. The important point is that when qualities are arranged in a series and identified with numbers, the use of those numbers to perform calculations like averages or percentages is meaningless, as the relationship between points 1 and 2, and between 5 and 6 in the series, may be completely different. Distinctions between qualitative entities can very often only be expressed through descriptions like 'more and less' or 'better and worse' as they have no true numerical meaning.

The third way in which numbers are used, is to describe quantitative relationships between things. Examples here might be weights or distances, or amounts of things. If we take one bag of sugar to weigh 1 unit and balance a similar bag of sugar opposite it so that neither bag sinks, we can say that the second bag also weighs 1 unit. We can then take a bigger bag of sugar and balance it against the two smaller bags, such that neither side sinks, and say that the bigger bag weighs 2 units. In this way we can construct a scale of measurement for the bags of sugar. This use of numbers is appropriate for properties that are additive. It applies to the quantitative analysis of scientific research, such as the measurement of blood pressure or blood levels of a drug or cholesterol. Unlike the case of the series, the distances between the points on these scales are equal and, therefore, we can construct measurements of means with standard deviations and talk of scales and percentages with meaning.

Scales and qualitative research

But what if the subject of the measurement is not an additive entity? For instance, can the degree of patient satisfaction with a doctor or of quality of life be described using a scale? Most qualitative research does not deal with qualities that are additive, so what are the problems of employing scales as a method of presenting its results? There are four main ones:

1. Ensuring that it is the same quality that is being measured from the highest to the lowest points on the scale.

2. Making the quality continuum explicit, i.e. is it possible to distinguish between discrete points along it?

3. Establishing 'the equality of differences', i.e. that each point on a scale is the same distance from another.

4. The effect of the observer on the construction of the scale and the measurements taken by it.

1. This problem can be illustrated by a study on doctors modes of dress.[29] The researchers acknowledged that they might not be measuring the patients' reactions to the pictures of doctors presented to them in the study but rather attitudes based on what the patients were used to in their own doctors. It is particularly when a respondent expresses an extreme view that the attitude under consideration may turn into something different. In this example, extreme disapproval of a casual mode of dress may reflect a personal dislike of wearing jeans, rather than any view as to what it is appropriate for a doctor to wear.

2. The second problem is whether it is possible to distinguish between discrete degrees of a quality along its continuum. Unless this can be done it is impossible to use numbers in any way, even as labels, as each point has to be clearly distinguishable from the next. Likert[30] encountered this problem in his description of a scale for the measurement of attitudes. His method depended on the construction of a statement to which people of different points of view would respond differentially according to the strength of their view from 'strongly approve' to 'strongly disapprove'. He gave an example of American attitudes toward

Japan. A more appropriate example for the UK currently might be attitudes towards Europe. In a referendum on closer integration with Europe, a statement like 'Britain should follow Germany's lead and favour complete integration with Europe' is likely to produce a predominantly negative response. It is difficult to think of a statement that would accurately reflect the spread of opinion on this subject, but suggesting that Britain should follow Germany's lead certainly would not. Likert scales are in common use in qualitative research[31] and great care needs to be taken in the construction of the statements employed, particularly if the researcher is constructing a scale of four or more points.

3. This problem involves ensuring that the discrete points are at equal numerical distances from each other:

> We must be on guard against a common error. It is often believed that because we can assign numbers to different degrees of a quality, the different degrees will always bear to each other the same ratio as do the numbers we have assigned to them. This is a serious mistake, and arises because it is supposed that measurement requires nothing more than the assigning of numbers.[32]

From the preceding consideration of numbers and their use it seems that the distinction between the second use (that of numbers arranged in a series) and the third (that of numbers to make quantitative distinctions) has become disregarded in some qualitative research. As an example of this, as part of a study looking at quality of care in general practice in Australia, Winefield *et al.*[33] measured doctor's satisfaction with a consultation using a visual analogue rating scale with points ranging from 0 = completely unsatisfying, to 5 = average in satisfaction, up to 10 = completely satisfying. The result of this analysis was expressed as a mean score of 8.95. This kind of method is valid in as much as it uses numbers in the first and second senses: both as labels to stand for certain doctor responses and as a method of placing responses in a series, such that a score of 1 is considered less satisfying than a score of 2. However, this method does not establish a *scale* for the measurement of satisfaction, as we cannot say that the amount of satisfaction between a score of 0 and 1 is the same as that distinguishing a score of 2 from that of 3. To express the scores as a mean presupposes the establishment of a scale and is, therefore, invalid.

4. This problem deals with the effect of the researcher on the construction of the scale and its use in measurement. In quantitative research, measurement and the use of scales is straightforward. The scales used are generally well established and are not dependent on the factor being researched. If we want to measure blood pressure, for instance, the mercury sphygmomanometer exists and all that need concern us is the precision of the reading taken by the observer. The measurement is objective as the instrument has not been devised by those carrying out the research. This is qualified, however, by the fact that in all measurement we do not just measure x but rather the situation that combines x and the effect of the measuring instrument y. Thus with the case of blood pressure measurement we may not get a result that is the true blood pressure (x) but rather a reading (xy), which is different because of an error made by the observer or the measuring instrument.

In qualitative research, the margin for such error is much greater as the researcher is himself often one of the research instruments. Because qualitative research aims to 'study things in their natural settings',[34] methods of measurement may have to be devised specifically for the quality under consideration in the context in which it appears. As an example of this, Law and Britten[35] use a method of measuring patient-centredness devised by Henbest and Stewart[36] to assess doctors' consulting styles. The measurement is based on scoring doctors on the basis of their response to a 'patient offer', i.e. anything the patient says that is of potential significance. If a doctor does not respond, he scores 0; if he responds with a closed question, he scores 1; if he allows the patient further expression, he scores 2; and if he actively facilitates the patient's expression, he scores 3. Audiotapes of the consultations were used for analysis.

But in this study, the researchers were the most significant factor in the resulting score xy (which combines the effect of the instrument, y, with what is measured, x), as they were the ones who were analysing the audiotaped consultations and deciding on scores. Thus, the researchers using this tool would listen to everything the doctor said as a reflection of his patient-centredness, and silence would score 0. But, in the true situation, silence might reflect the fact that the doctor knew the patient very well and might not need to say anything or might need only to touch the patient's hand to encourage them to express their concerns more fully. Even if the researcher were directly observing the doctor–patient interaction, he would be interpreting the doctor's response for the scoring system. Would he count a smile from the doctor as active facilitation of the patient's expression or not? The main point is that the measurement tool might distort what is being measured and may turn a positive response into something negative.

There are, therefore, problems both with establishing that qualitative analysis is amenable to the use of scales at all, never mind whether numbers can be used in that analysis. Even when numbers are used in a series, it is important to indicate their direction, e.g. that 1 represents very satisfied and 5 very dissatisfied, rather than the other way round. This is entirely at the discretion of the researcher and reflects how meaningless as numbers these labels are. Letters of the alphabet could just as easily be used, except that they are limited to a series of 26. The judgement of the researcher is paramount, and the attempt to disguise this by appealing to numbers is unconvincing.

The conclusion of this discussion is that the results of qualitative research cannot satisfactorily be quantified. They cannot because of the nature of the subjects under consideration (i.e. subjects such as doctor or patient attitudes); because the research is context-specific (i.e. describes a particular hospital clinic or general practice); and because of the researcher influence on the measurement process. It follows from this conclusion that we cannot use the procedures of scientific induction to generalize these results; and if they cannot be generalized, how can they be of benefit to clinicians? All research aims at increasing our understanding, but for *clinical* research to be worthwhile, it additionally needs to produce some lessons for wider clinical practice. Can qualitative research do this? This takes us to the second question: granted that qualitative research cannot use scales, is it scientific?

Generalizability and qualitative research: a route to understanding

In considering the question whether qualitative research can be considered scientific, even if it is not quantitative, we shall refer back to our original characterization of science (Section 1.2.1). It seems clear that qualitative research can satisfy some, but not all, of these criteria. Thus, it clearly involves observation, the recording of these observations, perhaps the use of 'instruments', such as video recorders, (even if not 'experimentation'), observation of the effects produced by the phenomenon under consideration (such as the effect of the doctor on the patient), the formation of hypotheses about causation, observation over a period of time, and no doubt others. We have suggested that where qualitative research goes wrong is in its attempt to adapt itself to other aspects of science, such as measurement, with the reductivism that this entails. Thus, in order to try to generate measurement, 'patient-centredness' (for example) becomes reduced to, or defined in terms of, a few operations, such as 'making eye contact'. But, as we have seen, qualitative research cannot satisfy the measurement criterion. Can it satisfy the generalizability criterion? This is more important, since generalizability, as we have suggested (Section 1.2.2) is perhaps a necessary, if not a sufficient, condition of the scientific. And it is certainly a necessary condition of qualitative research being useful to clinicians.

The qualitative researcher cannot generalize by means of the usual procedures of scientific generalization—induction from a range of relevantly similar instances. He cannot do this because, as we have seen, induction, in the clinical situation, requires the researcher to ignore the many complexities of human encounters and concentrate on only a few. How then, if at all, can the qualitative researcher generalize? The lessons of qualitative research for clinicians are derived from considering the plausibility of the particular situation in terms of their own and on finding parallels that are helpful. The question for the reader of this material is, 'Are there any universal features in this situation that I recognize and can apply?'. Understanding in qualitative research is, therefore, more akin to the understanding gained from an art or, perhaps, philosophy, rather than from a numerical science. This does not mean that it is an inferior kind of understanding, but it does mean that it is different in that it is reached by a different route. It requires the active participation of the reader to identify with the situation and relate the findings to his own situation.

Consider the following example from Sartre.[37] Sartre describes a man bending down to listen at a keyhole. He believes his wife is in the room with her lover. Suddenly he hears a step behind him, and immediately his attitude changes. To begin with, he wanted to hear a conversation, but now he has become an object to someone else—an eavesdropper to be described and despised. Sartre uses the example to show how we cannot think of ourselves as separate from others. But we could also use it to show that moral emotions, such as shame, are experienced in a social context. The eavesdropper minds being caught, not for any utilitarian-type reasons, but because he must now think of himself as mean and sneaky. He despises such characteristics in others and now he must despise himself. This constitutes shame.

We have used this example because it is similar to many in qualitative medical research. The route to understanding is through our identification with the situation to universal features of human emotions. There is an element of generalization, but not by induction. The imposition of quantitative language obstructs this understanding by distorting the findings of qualitative research and making them obscure to the reader. Even if the approach of such research is narrative and descriptive of particular situations it is still aiming at providing understanding of general features of clinical situations. In presenting its results it might, therefore, do well to follow the example of philosophy and guide judgement by using words. Qualitative researchers take pride in the fact that their approach provides new insight into clinical situations. They should not hide these insights under a numerical bushel but illuminate it with language that reflects the new kind of understanding they wish to convey.

In sum, then, is qualitative research scientific? We have claimed that the activities of science make up a large family. Qualitative research has some of the family characteristics, but it gives generalized understanding by a different route. The judgement of the researcher is all-important in this kind of research.

1.7.4 Clinical trials

Awareness in medical circles that much medical research on treatments did not meet the strong criteria of proof demanded by the natural sciences led investigators to seek statistical techniques that would establish degrees of confidence for the conclusions of empirical studies. The idea is a simple one. If a form of treatment is of uncertain value, or if there is doubt about which of two treatments is the better, patients are randomized to one or other, and the outcome is assessed by statistical methods. There are refinements called 'double-blind studies' in which neither the patient nor the doctor administering the treatment know who has been given the drug and who the inert substance. There are further refinements called 'cross-over studies' in which following a period with drug A the patient is switched to drug B. Cross-over studies can also be double-blind. Our concern here, however, is not with the detailed technicalities of clinical trials but with the question of their scientific status. It must also be stressed that settling the question of the scientific status of clinical trials does not in itself settle the question of the effectiveness of treatments in a clinical examination with a patient. A drug that a trial has pronounced efficacious might not be effective with a given patient. Indeed, a drug that a trial has declared to be non-efficacious might still be effective with a given patient in a clinical examination. This issue we shall discuss in the next chapter and concentrate for the moment on the scientific status of clinical trials.

There is no doubt that the RCT is widely regarded as one of the most important developments in medical research in the last 50 years and it has been applied widely to the study of treatments in almost every area of medical practice. It is thought to provide the basis for 'evidence-based medicine' and as such it is regarded in medical research as the 'gold standard'. And it certainly satisfies some of the criteria for science. Thus it involves observation, the recording of observations, observation of the effects produced by the phenomenon under consideration (such as the effect of a drug on a disease), perhaps the formation of hypotheses about causation, and, certainly, observation over a period of time. Unlike qualitative research, it can undoubtedly use numbers, since it is avowedly reductivist as it deals just with, for example, drugs and diseases, and discounts the human factors. But purely as science it suffers from a large defect. In discussing the nature of science we suggested that scientific endeavour is directed at systematic understanding. It is systematic understanding that, as Smith says (Section 1.6) 'soothes the imagination'. But what the RCT offers is *at best* a statistical probability that a treatment will work. The judgements of researchers are necessary to advise on whether the probability is significant or not. We say *at best* for it has been argued that even beginning a study changes the outcome of the condition studied, probably because of the greater care and interest shown by the research team.[38] What we find in the RCT is science in the Baconian sense of empirical studies of what might 'work' in a statistically significant set of cases. As we have seen, however, the activities that might be regarded as 'scientific' make up a large family. In terms of the family metaphor the RCT is a cousin!

While it might be a 'gold standard' in estimating the efficacy of treatments, the RCT is hardly a gold standard in science. It is at the 'natural history' end of science in that it is recording correlations without purporting to offer any causal understanding of why they are correlated. But true science, as Smith says, seeks the connecting principles of nature, rather than what seems to work in some cases.

Currently the idea of 'meta-analysis' is fashionable. But this complex kind of systematic review of research studies does not avoid the problems we raise. For example, judgement (and complex judgement) is required to decide on the comparability of the studies in the meta-analysis. In fact, meta-analysis may simply create new possibilities for error by compounding the errors of the original studies. The judgement of the researchers is all-important here to interpret the results. The cynical might fear that these researchers do not always have the detachment, impartiality, and rigour of the true scientist (Section 1.2), since the need to 'get results', please funding bodies, and publish papers may at times distort judgement.

1.8 Is medical research scientific?

We began by distinguishing three different sorts of medical research:

(1) into the normal and pathological workings of the body;

(2) observational studies, which we divided into simple and complicated descriptive quantitative studies, and qualitative studies of the behaviour of patients, doctors and their interactions;

(3) experimental studies, such as randomized trials, which involve an intervention.

It emerged that (1) is clearly scientific, whereas (2) and (3) are much more doubtfully so. What are the basic differences between (1), and (2) and (3)? There are two basic points of differences that explain why (1) is true science, whereas (2) and (3) are on the fringes, are cousins of science.

The first is that science, by its very nature, is reductionist. The scientist must isolate the phenomena to be investigated. Galileo or Newton, for example, concentrate on the primary or measurable qualities of matter, or employ idealizations such as 'frictionless plane'. The basic medical sciences—biochemistry, etc.—are similarly reductionist. They can, therefore, work effectively as sciences. But (2) is concerned with actual human behaviour and the reductionist attempt here—in the use of scales, for example—is bound to fail. Research of this kind is based on holistic assumptions, and the use of reductionist quantitative methods can produce only distorted results or half-truths. Turning now to (3), the RCT, we find that it too attempts to use reductionist quantitative methods. The methods are reductionist in that they are abstracting from the complexities of actual clinical encounters. For example, they totally ignore the greatest asset of medical practice—the doctor–patient relationship. Once again, half-truths are all that emerge, and moreover half-truths without any systematic basis.

The second reason why (2) and (3), but not (1), are not fully scientific is that (1), like true science, is driven by concerns internal to the investigations, whereas (2) and (3) are driven by goals external to the investigation, such as the search for efficacious treatments. In the words of Bacon, 'Truth therefore and utility are here the very same thing'.[39] But such an attitude is not that of the scientist searching for the systematic under-standing provided by the 'connecting principles of nature'.

1.9 Judgement in medical research

The fact that 'medical research' comprises a variety of activities means that the need for judgement by the researcher will also vary. We have argued that, even in the areas of research that exhibit the paradigm features of science, personal judgement is essential, for example, in assessing the relevance and weight to place on the evidence-base. But when we look at the scientific cousins of the core activities, we find that the judgement of the researcher is absolutely central. Indeed, in the case of qualitative research, the insights and interpretations of the researcher are better seen as analogous to the judgements of the literary critic than to those of the biologist. It is quite misleading to attempt to quantify such judgement. Even in the alleged 'gold standard' RCTs, we find a central need for judgement to interpret the results. In all cases we may hope that the judgements of the researchers will be detached, impartial, and as rigorous as the subject-matter permits. That is why any fear of commercial or other bias is very disturbing.

Scientific or technical judgement so understood is one component of good clinical judgement, but it is not yet 'evidence in practice'. To understand that we must turn to the clinical situation.

1.10 Conclusions

1. Science can be characterized in terms of a method, a certain use of evidence, and an aim.
2. The method is complex but involves observation, hypothesis formation, and further experiments. Evidence has a par-ticular logical place in scientific method.

3. The aim of science is primarily to achieve a particular sort of systematic understanding, although there is also an empirical, Baconian tradition, which sees the aim of science as utility.

4. Science involves the imagination, which is stimulated by irregularities and satisfied by wider systems.

5. Medical research involves:
   (a) basic biology and pathology;
   (b) observational studies, including quantitative research of both a simple descriptive sort and also more complicated patient population studies, and qualitative research;
   (c) RCTs.

   Central scientific demands are fulfilled in (a), but (b) and (c) are in different ways on the periphery of science.

6. In all areas of medical research the judgement of the researcher is necessary, especially in 5(b) and 5(c).

References

1. Lerner L, ed. *Evidence and Inference.* Illinois: the Free Press of Glencoe, 1959, p.13.
2. Hempel C, Studies in the Logic of Confirmation in Achinstein P. ed. *The Concept of Evidence.* Oxford: Oxford University Press, 1983, p.12.
3. Conan Doyle A, *A Study in Scarlet and the Sign of Four.* London: Elder and Co., 1903, p.39.
4. Hempel op. cit., p.14.
5. Lerner op. cit., p.13.
6. Koestler A, *Insight and Outlook.* London : Macmillan and Co. Ltd., 1949, p.252.
7. Bacon Francis, *Advancement of Learning* (1605), ed. J Devey, London: Bell, 1872, Bk. I.
8. Bacon Francis, *Novum Organum* (1620), ed. J Devey, London: Bell, 1872, Bk. I, sect. 1.
9. Bacon Francis, 1620 op. cit. Bk. I, sect. 129.
10. Bacon Francis, 1620 op. cit. Bk. I, sect. 124.
11. Smith A, (1740–46) History of astronomy. Collected in *The Scottish Enlightenment* (ed. A Broadie) Edinburgh: Canongate Classics, 1997, pp. 735–49,
12. Smith, op. cit., p.735.
13. Smith, op. cit., p.747.
14. Smith, op. cit., p.747.
15. Bonelllie SR, Raab GM. Why are babies getting heavier? Comparison of Scottish births from 1980 to 1992. *BMJ* 1999; 315: 1205.

16. Meier C, Derby L, Jick S, Vasilakis C, Jick H, Antibiotics and risk of subsequent first-time acute myocardial infarction. *Journal of the American Medical Association (JAMA)* 1999: 281; 427–31. See p. 417 News *BMJ* 13 Feb 1999.

17. Doll R, Peto R, Weatley K, Gray R, Sutherland I, Mortality in relation to smoking: 40 years' observations on male British doctors. *BMJ* 1994: 309: 901–11.

18. Farmer R, Miller D, Lawrenson R. *Lecture Notes on Epidemiology and Public Health Medicine*, 4th edn. Oxford: Blackwell, 1996. p.51.

19. Macnaughton RJ, Numbers, scales and qualitative research. *Lancet* 1996; 347: 1099–1100.

20. Jones R. Why do qualitative research? *BMJ* 1995; 131:2 And following series of articles.

21. Britten N, Jones R, Murphy E, Stacey R, Qualitative research methods in general practice and primary care. *Family Practice* 1995; 12: 104–114.

22. Sylvester S, General practitioners' attitudes to professional reacreditation. *BMJ* 1993; 307: 912–14.

23. Kinmonth A, Understanding and meaning in research and practice. *Family Practice* 1995; 12: 1–2.

24. Law SAT, Britten N, Factors that influence the patient-centredness of a consultation. *British Journal of General Practice (BJGP)* 1995; 45:520–24.

25. Winefield HR, Murrell TG, Clifford J, Process and outcomes in general practice consultations: problems in defining high quality care. *Social Science and Medicine* 1995; 41: 969–75.

26. Mays N, Pope C, Rigour and qualitative research. *BMJ* 1995; 311: 109–12.

27. Nagel E, Measurement. In *Philosophy of Science* (ed. Danto A, Morgenbesser S). Cleveland: Meridian books, 1960 p. 121.

28. Cohen MR, Nagel E, *An Introduction to Logic and Scientific Method*. London: Routledge and Kegan Paul Ltd., 1934, p. 294.

29. McKinstry B, Wang J, Putting on the style: what patients think of the way their doctor dresses. *BJGP* 1991; 41:275–78.

30. Likert R, A technique for the measurement of attitudes. *Archives of Psychology* 1932; 140: 1–55.

31. Peacock JL, Bland JM, Anderson HR, Pretem delivery: effects of socioeconomic factors, psychological stress, alcohol and caffeine. *BMJ* 1995; 311: 531–35.

32. Cohen and Nagel, op. cit., p.294.

33. Winefield *et al.*, op. cit.

34. Britten *et al.*, op. cit.

35. Law and Britten, op. cit.

36. Henbest RJ, Stewart MA, Patient-centredness in the consultation. 1: a method for measurement. *Family Practice* 1989; 6: 249–253.

37. Sartre J-P, *Being and Nothingness* (1943) trans. by Hazel E Barnes. London: Methuen, 1969. pp. 259–263.

38. Lyons B, Sugden R, Weale A. Organisations. In: *The Theory of Choice: a Critical Appraisal* (ed. Heap S, Hollis M *et al.*). Oxford: Blackwell, 1994. pp. 167–68.

39. Bacon Francis 1620, op. cit. Bk. I, sect. 73 and Bk. I, sect. 124.

2 Judgement in the clinic

2.1 Introduction

We have argued that if we adopt a broad interpretation of 'science' we can assert that all medical research is in some sense scientific, or evidence-based, although not necessarily quantitative. It follows from this that the research base of clinical practice is scientific in a broad sense. It does not follow, however, that clinical practice itself is, or indeed ought to be, fully scientific or evidence-based. If medical research is 'science', our question in this chapter is: To what extent is a clinical consultation simply a matter of applying that science? It will emerge that there is much more to the consultation, or to good clinical practice, than simply applying science, or applying the evidence, to a given patient. Our discussion will be concerned with the extent and nature of the 'much more'.

It is a commonplace to say in this kind of context that the 'much more' consists in just this: that clinical medicine is an 'art'. We do not dissent from this, but those who take it as obvious, as a cliché, that clinical medicine is an art, rarely go on to specify what that means or consists in. Just as in our last chapter we were concerned to analyse in some detail the equally familiar claim that medicine is a science, so in this chapter we shall be concerned with spelling out, in critical detail, what it means to say that clinical medicine is an art. It will emerge once again that a particular sort of judgement is involved.

There are, of course, differences between different medical specialties in respect of the proportion of science and art, but basically the difference between medical research and clinical practice is this: medical research is concerned with providing generalized, systematic understanding, or at least with discovering statistically significant correlations, whereas clinical practice is concerned with establishing the diagnosis, prognosis, and treatment of individual human beings who happen to have illnesses, diseases, injuries, or other maladies. The question then arises: How far can the inherent reductivism of scientific research be adapted to the holism of the individual consultation? More simply, we are asking: How far does evidence-based medicine fit in with the central activities of clinical practice during consultations? What is the balance between evidence and humane judgement?

2.2 A clinical example

The doctor who has listened to a patient's account of what is wrong and is faced with research evidence of treatments will, in the end, make a judgement about the best course to follow for the patient. What are the components in this clinical judgement? The good doctor, the one (as we shall see in Chapter 3) who has a 'humane attitude', will see the need: to individualize the generalized evidence; to listen to the patient's stories about the origins of their problems; to interpret these stories and gain insight in to the root of the problems; and to obtain consent for any proposed treatment. We shall show in Chapter 3 how all these requirements for a good consultation relate to humane understanding and judgement.

But in this chapter we shall consider how generalized evidence is individualized; how 'anecdotes' or stories are relevant to the clinician, but require interpretation; and what consent means to the good clinician. This can best be illustrated in an example of a consultation.

Consultations may be classified in different ways: behaviour orientated models emphasize the doctor's activities,[1, 2] whereas task-orientated models suggest a series of predefined activities to be completed.[3] We will use the task-based approach of Pendleton[4]—a model applicable to hospital and general practice—to assess the kinds of evidence used by doctors at various stages during the consultation. Our fictitious patient is Mrs Mackay, a 70-year-old widow who suffers from osteoarthritis and non-insulin-dependent diabetes (NIDDM).[5]

Mrs Mackay has been recently widowed and now frequently attends her general practitioner's surgery. Following the Pendleton model, the doctor's first task is to explore Mrs Mackay's ideas and concerns about her symptoms and to discover what she expects the outcome of the consultation to be. On this occasion, Mrs Mackay complains of dizziness and appears to be very anxious about this symptom. The important evidence during this stage of the consultation is the patient's story and her associated behaviour.[6] Exploration of Mrs Mackay's concerns, ideas, and expectations allows the doctor to discover what conclusion the patient has drawn about her symptoms. Thus the doctor can tap into the patient's health beliefs and the sources of these beliefs. These sources can be diverse and include anecdotal evidence from family, friends, family traditions, television programmes, and magazine and newspaper articles. Mrs Mackay believes that dizziness means that her blood pressure may be high; her experience with her husband (who had hypertension and died from a stroke) tells her that she is at risk of imminent death or disability, and she is therefore anxious.

The doctor's second task is to consider the reason for attendance in sufficient detail to reach a diagnosis before moving on to review any other difficulties and risk factors. Scientific evidence has a greater role here than in the preliminary discussion with the patient. Mrs Mackay's blood pressure is, indeed, high (170/100 mmHg) and this is the third time it has been raised. Has there been any renal damage associated with her diabetes? Are there any other underlying factors, such as alcohol abuse or depression? The doctor then reviews Mrs Mackay's glycaemic control and discovers that at the most recent measurement of glycosylated haemoglobin (HbA1c, a measure of blood sugar levels over the preceding 3 months), the concentration was raised.

The doctor's third task is to chose an appropriate action for the problem. Here the doctor must consider the evidence on the specific clinical problem (in this case hypertension) and that relating to the individual patient. According to the rules of evidence-based medicine, Mrs Mackay needs treatment and one option for a woman of her age is a thiazide diuretic.[7] Mrs Mackay is at risk of stroke but she also has NIDDM and is taking an oral hypoglycaemic agent; her diabetes has been poorly controlled since her husband's death. Should the doctor put Mrs Mackay at further risk by prescribing another medication that might interfere with her glycaemic control? Mrs Mackay has osteoarthritis and poor mobility; will increased diuresis exacerbate her problems? On the other hand, Mrs Mackay believes that high blood pressure leads to stroke, and from what the doctor knows of this patient, any additional anxiety during her bereavement might make it difficult for her to cope. The decision to use the evidence in the context of the consultation is a matter for clinical judgement; the doctor must think about the patient's multiple pathology and drug treatments, and, most importantly, whether any new treatment is acceptable to the patient herself.

The doctor's fourth task is to ensure mutual understanding between doctor and patient and shared acceptance of the selected further action or treatment. The doctor must, therefore, move towards the patient's own unscientific view.

The final task is for the doctor to establish and maintain a therapeutic relationship with the patient. Such a relationship is tremendously beneficial for the patient; indeed the placebo effect of the 'drug doctor' cannot be easily assessed by an evidence-based approach.

From the example of Mrs Mackay we can analyse what evidence is available during the consultation. The primary, and most important, source of evidence for clinical decision-making is the information that Mrs Mackay communicates verbally and non-verbally. The doctor's pre-existing knowledge of the patient is supplemented by medical records—available information includes not only the formal medical history and examination, but results of investigations.

The most important perception filter is the doctor's undergraduate studies. The knowledge, skills and attitudes of doctors reflect the medical orthodoxy at the time of their qualification. This wisdom diminishes after the final exams[8] and may not be updated with new information. In addition, much of the evidence taught in postgraduate courses is of limited value to the practitioners at whom it is directed.[9] Many doctors read the available medical literature for up to four hours per week[10] but even the most dedicated practitioner cannot critically appraise and assimilate the deluge of evidence published on a daily or weekly basis. Furthermore, much of the evidence is hard to find, or is outdated, or simply wrong.[11] To each of these formal types of evidence might be added clinical experience—which may be direct or indirect—from cases discussed with colleagues and reviews in case-series, clinical trials, or individual case-studies.

Current theories about how professionals integrate this diverse evidence into the routines of their daily practice suggest that doctors become more expert in the use of evidence in consultations by remembering what has been termed the 'illness scripts' of previous patients.[12] This theory explains how clinical experience and the ability to learn from those experiences can modify clinical expertise and practice. Information about the current case is compared with similar cases stored in the doctor's long-term memory. The doctor uses this comparison to make a diagnosis and assess the outlook for the patient. When Mrs Mackay's illness script deviates from those with which the doctor is familiar, the resulting uncertainty may lead to a decision to seek further evidence or refer the patient to a colleague whom the doctor believes has greater experience of this type of problem.

The analysis of this fictional consultation does not give prominence to the practice of evidence-based medicine. Rather, the doctor seems to apply a sliding scale of importance to the evidence from different sources that depends on the specific illness and the patient.

Scientific evidence should come from the most valid and reliable source, which is usually up-to-date, peer-reviewed papers. New rapid means of information delivery should provide the doctor with just enough information for them to make a judgement appropriate to each patient in the limited time available during consultations. However, the evidence itself is no substitute for clinical judgement; evidence must still be interpreted and applied to the individual patient. For example, in autumn 1995, there was controversy about the combined oral contraceptive pill:[13] doctors objected because they had been given the conclusions derived from the studies concerned before the studies themselves were published and available for scrutiny.

This meant that the full details were not provided for them to judge whether the data applied to individual patients.

Furthermore, an evidence-based approach views the evidence from randomized, controlled trials as the most valid. However, in the consultation, the doctor deals with an individual patient. The results of randomized, controlled trials that involve large numbers of participants may not be applicable to a specific case.[14] As we argued in Section 1.7.4, randomized, controlled trials produce an oversimplified and artificial environment, which may bear little resemblance to day-to-day reality. Indeed, even when the evidence is good, it does not necessarily have to be applied. Other important factors, not least of which is that the patient may not wish to take the treatment, need to be considered.

Evidence-based medicine constructs a hierarchy[15] with randomized, controlled trials at the top and evidence from clinical experience, or shared stories about other doctors' patients, at the bottom. The above analysis of consultation tasks suggests that at times experimental, and at times anecdotal, evidence will be the most important parts of understanding the patient's condition and implementing treatment through a good doctor–patient relationship. The decision about what kind of evidence is the most important is a matter for clinical judgement.

Evidence-based medicine can benefit medical practice because it will help ensure that all patients have access to the most up-to-date and well-validated evidence through their doctors. However, patients are not clones and doctors are not automatons. All patients differ subtly in their presentation of illness, in their understanding and acceptance of medical advice, and in their response to treatment. Doctors need to know the latest research but should apply new advances with judgement and an awareness of the unique circumstances of the individual patient's case. Information technology has helped to make evidence available from a variety of sources during the consultation. Science, however, is unlikely ever to be able to make all the necessary distinctions required to answer all the questions that patients bring to their doctors. Medicine will always require thoughtful doctors who are able to filter the evidence appropriate to each patient through an individualized approach. Let us consider further the nature of individualized evidence.

2.3 Individualized evidence

2.3.1 The detective model

Scientists are not the only professionals to be interested in evidence. Detectives, for example, are interested in evidence.[16] As we have seen (Section 1.3.1), the role of the detective, as suggested by Sherlock Holmes, is to amass all the material relating to a case and then formulate some hypothesis as to its solution. We have argued that Holmes has a different view of the relationship between evidence and hypothesis from that of the scientist, but there is another important difference, relevant to our present clinical concerns, between the scientific and the detective model of evidence.

Let us imagine that the Duke is found murdered in the library. The investigating detective takes statements from many people—other family members, maids, gardeners and the butler. These statements are the data concerning the case. The detective then formulates the hypothesis that it was the Duchess's lover who committed the crime. The information relating to the lover's involvement then turns into evidence because it relates to a particular hypothesis in the case. However, the detective then turns up a convincing piece of counter-evidence: an alibi for the lover. A new hypothesis must then be formulated—that the culprit was in fact the butler. And so the process goes on.

This 'detective model' of evidence is similar to the scientific model in important respects—the collection of data, the observations, the chance discoveries, followed by the formulation of hypotheses, which transform some of this information into evidence and suggest how other evidence (for or against the hypotheses) might be found. But it is unlike the scientific model in at least this important respect: it is not logically possible to generalize. The evidence is relevant to one and only one situation. Both the scientific and the detective models have truth as their goal, but in the one case it is general truth, and in the other it is truth specific to a situation. This is an important difference and it is one that highlights the need for judgement. Moreover, the nature of the insight involved seems not unlike that in the scientific model, for it requires the sifting and evaluation of information and findings, and the relating of these to hypotheses. Once again, this sort of judgement requires technical knowledge.

2.3.2 Medical evidence

Let us now look at the application of these models to the medical context. Does the use of evidence and judgement in medicine have more in common with the work of a detective or with that of a scientist? It might seem that medicine uses both models. On the one hand, the work of clinical *research* involves rigorous application of the science model to clinical problems. The aim of research studies is to establish truths about clinical diagnosis and treatment, which will be true for all common situations. It might also seem that, on the other hand, if we look at the work of clinical *practice*, the work of the individual doctor in the surgery or clinic, this has more in common with the work of the detective. The taking of a clinical history parallels the taking of statements of witnesses to a crime and the examination process is like the rigorous examination of the crime scene. The doctor is here amassing unstructured data, which he will then use to suggest a diagnosis (the hypothesis) and will attempt to establish the truth of that diagnosis by further examination (through X-rays, laboratory testing of blood samples, etc.). These two kinds of activity are quite different but they have this in common: both are concerned with discussing truth, the general-ized truth of science or the specific truth of diagnosis, and both involve a similar sort of technical judgement.

Clinical practice, however, has two aspects to it: diagnosis (and for present purposes we can include prognosis under this heading) and treatment. Now, of course, the proponents of evidence-based medicine will correctly say that it is precisely at the point of treatment that scientific evidence is relevant, that it is a matter of scientific truth that some treatments are more effective than others. But the clinician is not concerned with treatments in the abstract. The clinician is concerned with treating *this* specific patient, and the treating of patients (as distinct from 'evidence-based treatments') requires the clinician to be influenced by many factors other than truth, such as the consent of this patient, the meaning of the disease for this patient, how important the side-effects are for this patient, whether this patient has heard of the treatment, family support, and perhaps even the cost. These factors have nothing to do with truth, whether general or specific. This point about the aim of clinical treatment leads us to propose a third model for evidence as it is used in medicine. This model involves a different sort of judgement, which is peculiar to clinical treatment.

2.3.3 A model of evidence in clinical medicine

This third model we will call the 'treatment' model of evidence. Kathryn Montgomery Hunter described the patient as:

...provid[ing] the text that medicine must read and make sense of and explain.[17]

She focuses on the importance of the individual patient as the primary source of evidence that the doctor requires to assess in the light of the presenting complaint. The process does not stop there, as it might in the context of detection or science, as the doctor must then initiate treatment appropriate, not only to the specific condition, but also to the specific patient. Doctors must, of course, have in their minds a knowledge of evidence-based treatments, but this part of the process also involves an assessment of other sorts of question: will the evidence relating to this patient suggest that they will be able to comply with treatment? Is it clear that the patient understands their condition and trusts the doctor's conclusion sufficiently for the benefits of the placebo effect to come into play? Is the treatment appropriate for the social situation of this patient?

For instance, evidence-based medicine might suggest that in mild to moderate acne, a topical antibiotic preparation is as effective as a course of oral antibiotics. But consider the case of Susie, a 17 year old who has recently started on the combined oral contraceptive pill and attends her doctor with acne, compared with that of Liz, a 21 year old presenting with the same problem, who is about to get married and is on a three monthly depot progesterone injection for contraception. Both have mild to moderate acne but Liz may wish to keep her face clear of medications on her forthcoming honeymoon and Susie needs to avoid oral antibiotics, which might interfere with her pill. In this case, therefore, social circumstances might dictate that Susie gets the application and Liz gets the tablets. However, if Susie declares that a friend of hers got antibiotic tablets and his acne disappeared 'like magic', the wise doctor would comply with the patient's desire and make use of the additional benefits that the patient's belief in the treatment might convey.

In the context of this model, we now see the paramount importance and peculiar nature of clinical judgement. We have seen how judgement is relevant to assessing relevance, weight, and drawing conclusions (Chapter 1), but it comes into its own when we deal with the range of complex factors in the clinical situation. This is a different sort of judgement and requires different abilities. The judgements of the scientist and the detective are technical; that of the clinician is based on what Aristotle calls *phronesis* or 'practical wisdom'.[18] It is certainly true that medicine is in some respects a *techne*, a skill-based activity,[19] whose practice requires the exercise of specific skills relating to diagnosis and treatment (see Section 3.2). It is in this sense that the judgements of medicine are like the technical ones of science and detective work, and relate to conclusions that are either true or false. But medicine involves more than this; it involves a 'capacity to act with regard to the things that are good or bad for man'.[20] When doctors have to come to a decision about treatments for individual patients—in other words, have to make judgements relating to 'the things that are good or bad for man'—this is not the same as making judgements about what is or is not the case. The insights of the consultation have more to do with what is or is not appropriate for this patient, with this condition, and at this time.

2.3.4 Provisional conclusion

There are several sorts of evidence each with its own correlative sort of insight or judgement. In the case of the medical scientist, the evidence comes from, say, randomized, controlled trials (Section 1.7.4), which suggest the percentage success or failure of treatments.[21] The correlative judgement is technical and is directed at generalized truth. It is often said that clinical treatment applies this scientific evidence to individual patients. This is certainly part of the picture; that part in which diagnostics is like detective work. The correlative judgements of the clinician are in this respect like those of the detective and aim at individualized truth about a given patient. But the other part of the clinical picture concerns treatment. Evidence about what constitutes the best treatment for a given patient involves a wide range of imponderables, but especially a patient's own (perhaps irrational) perspective. The correlative judgement in this case can be only partly technical (i.e. based on evidence-based treatments) because it must tap into the belief system of the patient and, indeed, of the doctor. These judgements do not aim at truth but at effective treatment. Hence, the judgements of the good clinician must be more than technical; they must show practical wisdom.

2.4 Anecdotes[22]

In the scientific, evidence-based atmosphere of contemporary medicine there is a tendency for doctors to believe that they can ignore the patient and concentrate on the disease, which they believe can be identified scientifically. The practice of ignoring the patient and concentrating on the disease is certainly ethically objectionable, but our concern here is that it is also neglecting an important source of information about the patient—the patient's own story. The patient may be telling the doctor what is wrong, but this kind of clinical evidence is often dismissed as 'anecdotal', where that term means that it is not worth bothering about. But we shall try to show in this section that anecdotes have an important function in the consultation, if not in the laboratory, and must be taken seriously by the good doctor.

2.4.1 What are anecdotes?

There appear to be two senses in which the word 'anecdote' is used. The first sense can be found in the sentence, 'And I would like to tell you an anecdote about this', and the second in, 'That's purely anecdotal'. The first sentence indicates the major sense of the word. The speaker is about to tell a short story illustrating a point he is wanting to make in a form that is more dramatic than merely stating the point. This introduction will frequently be followed by, 'I remember when I...' or 'I knew a man once who...', and the account may be fictional or non-fictional. In the medical context, anecdotes are largely non-fictional but in other contexts, such as in the world of stand-up comedy, they are often made up or may be reality embellished for effect. Many of the warning stories told to children are anecdotes of this latter type. For instance a mother might tell her child: 'I remember a little girl who once played too near the river and she fell in and was never found'. This anecdote briefly but dramatically illustrates the dangers of playing near the river. It may well be true that the mother knew a child who fell into the river but her death and disappearance are more likely to be embellishments calculated to make the story stick in her child's mind.

Another fruitful source of anecdotes is the obituary pages of the newspapers. Here is an extract from one of an English painter who died recently:

...though he had his moments of ready conviviality, he never really belonged to the art world. Possibly his personal background had something to do with this. He was born into a working-class family in Lancashire.... It is recorded that when his father asked him what he thought he wanted to do for a living, and he answered that he wanted to be a painter, his father was very happy, assuming that what he wanted to paint was houses.[23]

The obituary differs from biography in that it must give a brief account of the person's life with some (often rather flattering) reference to their character. Anecdotes are often included as memorable stories about the person's life, which also, as here, serve to illustrate or account for a trait of character. Here the painter's humble origins are told and the anecdote about his father's mistake serves to illustrate that those origins and upbringing were sufficiently strong to make him less inclined to join in with the parties and glamour of the art world.

The second sentence, 'That's purely anecdotal' gives a related but different sense of the word to the first. 'Anecdotal' information or evidence is information derived purely from anecdote and (as is usually implied) is not to be relied upon. It is not reliable because of the features that distinguish the anecdote: that it is a short, dramatic account, told for effect and liable to be embellished. The word 'anecdotage' has occasionally been used[24] to describe the activity of telling or making use of anecdote and its derogatory meaning is made all too clear by its relationship with 'dotage'. In medicine in particular, the term 'anecdotal' has developed a pejorative meaning, particularly so in recent times when doctors have been much concerned with evidence-based medicine. It is this recent emphasis that has been put on the scientific evidence base of medicine, which has led many authors to reassert the importance of other information, including stories[25] and anecdotes[26] as part of that evidence base. But, as we shall see in the following sections, anecdotes are an important source of treatments, diagnoses, and even therapy. Let us begin with doctor–doctor anecdotes as a source of treatments.

2.4.2 Doctor–doctor anecdotes

Anecdotes are told in all situations, formal and informal, where doctors get together. One good but trivial reason for this is that everyone enjoys a story. Stories enliven dull conference proceedings and serious medical meetings. The anecdotes told by doctors at these formal meetings can be lighthearted and aimed at lightening the atmosphere. More usually, the anecdote is told from the doctor's own experience for a good reason, and the telling of anecdotes is so much a part of communication between doctors that the teller may not even be consciously aware of that reason. Katherine Montgomery Hunter in her book *Doctors' Stories* underlines this point. Her book amounts to an anthropological study of 'doctors in the wild' and she sees the telling of anecdotes as instinctive medical behaviour. She characterizes the ideal environment for anecdote-telling in this way:

In general, it seems that the smaller and more regular the group, and the more its members are engaged in the same clinical activities, the more anecdotes will be told.[27]

The kind of setting described here is most likely to be a ward-round or hospital unit, or general practice case conference. But anecdotes are also told in formal settings, such as at conferences, hospital meetings, and in written form in journals. Usually the story has an illustrative function. At a conference presentation, alongside the scientific data on a new therapy, for example, a case may be cited as an example of how well the therapy worked. The cited case is usually one in which the therapy worked particularly well or, alternatively, a case in which the therapy was a complete failure. Anecdotes are generally dramatic stories and do not recount the commonplace, so these stories serve to illustrate the best and the worst of the therapy, and the audience are given the scientific evidence to assess as well. Anecdotes, in this setting, have a role in drawing the doctor's attention to the promise and pitfalls of new treatments when they are proposed.

In the discussion that follows a conference or case-conference presentation, the audience will often use anecdotes to provide counter-examples to what has been presented: 'Your patient may have responded in that way but I tried that in a patient of mine once and she nearly died'. Because anecdotes by their nature are memorable, one told by a speaker may stimulate the memory of another doctor in the audience and will produce a discussion on the usefulness of a therapy under a different set of circumstances in another patient.

These examples point to the value of anecdotes in continuing medical education as they provide real examples and counter-examples on which practising doctors can hone and test their medical knowledge, and keep it up to date. Such anecdote swapping also enables doctors to test their clinical judgement against that of their peers and sharpen it. But anecdotes are also in frequent use in undergraduate medical education. Clinical teaching in the wards goes on around the bed of a patient with a particular illness and clinical signs. Frequently, the clinician who is doing the teaching will make reference by anecdote to other similar cases that they have come across for comparison. Besides this, the teacher will also put forward hypothetical situations such as, 'What if this patient *had* had an MI? How would this change your management?'. These scenarios we might regard as hypothetical anecdotes and they serve to extend the educational value of the single case.

Anecdotes are often told to students about the great medical figures of the past, often to illustrate the importance of some very basic medical truth. One such example is a story told of the great Sir James Mackenzie, a general practitioner and pioneer in the field of cardiology in the early part of this century:

Mackenzie was making a weekend visit to his university city of Edinburgh. A surgeon invited him to give his opinion on the circulatory condition of a woman in a ward at the Infirmary, awaiting chole- cystectomy. She was found to have anomalous heart sounds. This had aroused doubt in the surgeon's mind about the wisdom of operating. The news of Mackenzie's visit had spread. A crowd of staff and students gathered in the ward. He talked to her about her home. It was on the top floor of a house in the Lawn Market. Did she shop for her family of six? Of course, who else? And carry it up the stairs? Indeed, yes. And how many times a day did she climb those stairs? Countless times. And did she find them trying? Why should she? Mackenzie turned to the surgeon and told him to operate with confidence so far as the function of the heart was concerned.[28]

This anecdote would reinforce the important medical maxim: 'Listen to the patient: they are giving you the diagnosis'.

As well as having a role in the education of current and future doctors, anecdotes help in the induction of doctors into the etiquette of the profession. Hospital residents, for instance, will seek advice from their predecessor on the preferred procedures in a new ward. Advice is frequently given in the form of an anecdote: 'Make sure you call the registrar the first time you do a lumbar puncture. I didn't and he tore strips off me for not checking with him first'.

Such professionalizing anecdotes are often of the warning type, 'Make sure you do this in case...' or 'Don't do that because...', but anecdotes can also provide a much needed support function. Medicine is not very good, as a profession, at providing formal support for practitioners when they have made mistakes or misjudgements. Case conferences and ward or practice meetings may provide this help often in the form of a supportive anecdote. A junior partner in our practice was upset at having missed a case of tuberculosis in a young slim patient with a cough. The senior partner responded: 'It is easily done. I did the same thing with a woman whom I thought was anorexic and then she suddenly coughed up blood and had to be rushed into hospital!' 'We've all done it' is an expression frequently heard when doctors admit their mistakes to their colleagues and what follows is an account of the other doctor's mistake, and reassurance that it can happen to us all. These supportive accounts do not just amount to crying on one another's shoulders, they usually lead to a shared learning experience. In the case of the TB misdiagnosis, the partners agreed to 'think TB' when dealing with persistent chest problems.

All the above functions of the anecdote occur through oral doctor–doctor communication. The written anecdote in the form of a single case report or 'A memorable patient' section, as in the *BMJ*, may serve an important function in stimulating investigation leading to new knowledge. Single case reports in the journals are often about puzzling cases that do not quite fit the prevailing scientific knowledge; it is such anomalies that serve to stimulate further research and discovery in medicine, particularly when doctors working in the same field find that they are picking up similar anomalies and a series of cases start to emerge. One famous example, cited by Dr Hunter, was the outbreak of phocomelia subsequently found to be associated with the anti-emetic, thalidomide, when used in pregnancy. A more recent example is the concern over the possible dangers of silicone breast implants, which have been raised by numerous anecdotal reports.[29] The anecdotes are not a substitute for systematic scientific research but they can point the research in the right direction in the first place.

We can see, therefore that doctor–doctor anecdotes can have a number of important functions: they draw attention to new medical treatments and diagnoses; they help hone medical knowledge and judgement; they have an important function in the education of current and future doctors; they assist the process of induction into the ways of the profession; and, finally, they may help to point research in a fruitful direction. They, therefore, have an important bearing on evidence and are factors in judgement.

2.4.3 Patient–doctor anecdotes

In the general practice setting, in particular, the patient's account of their problem is undifferentiated and unmedicalized because they have not yet had their story reinterpreted by a doctor. For instance, angina is not yet, 'A tight pain in my chest which I get with exertion'; it is still described in this way:

The reason I am here, doctor, is that last week I was walking to the shops with my wife and we came back with a lot of shopping and had to climb up the hill to the house because the bus broke down. As we reached the top of the hill I suddenly got this pain in my chest which made me stop and gasp for breath.

So anecdotes are often the way in which patients will explain their visit to the doctor in the first place.

Anecdotes are also used by patients to illustrate how the particular symptoms are affecting their lives at that time. This is an exchange one of the authors (JM) had with a patient who is particularly keen on the game of bowls:

JM: How are the knees just now? Are the new painkillers working better?

Patient: Oh no, it's just as bad, doctor, and with me Lady President of the bowling green this season too.

JM: How are you getting on with the bowling?

Patient: Oh, I'm not able to play just now. The last time I had a match I tried to deliver a bowl and I couldn't get up again! Some of the men had to lift me up off the green. It gave everyone a good laugh but I haven't been able to play since.

This kind of patient anecdote is important because it reflects the individual's experience of the problem and gives the doctor a clear idea of how function is affected. For the patient, mild osteoarthritis of the knees was having a major impact on her lifestyle and merited physiotherapy and an orthopaedic surgeon's opinion. For another elderly woman, whose lifestyle was not so active, the condition might not have prompted any action. The anecdote reminds us that what the patient is interested in is their ability to function, not the severity or otherwise of the pathology. Doctors will often say reassuringly to their patients, 'You'll be glad to hear that the test result is normal', only to be greeted with, 'So why am I having these problems?'. Patients want to be restored to normal function or at least to have an explanation for why they cannot function normally.

Patients' illustrative anecdotes can also be revealing of their understanding or misunderstanding of a suspected illness. A patient who had a urostomy scar that had developed a herniation commented:

But my Uncle James had his hernias operated on down here [indicating her groin area]. I thought it was only men that had hernias. Mind you my sister has one up here inside [indicating the epigastric area] and she has problems eating with it.

This series of anecdotes reveals the patient's (reasonable) confusion over the idea of a hernia and how it can exist in several different places. Paying attention to patient anecdote allows doctors the chance to clarify areas of misunderstanding and become aware of how the patient perceives their illness and their own ability to do something about it.

Even the way in which a patient orders events in her story can be highly significant. Compare two presentations of breast cancer:

About a month ago I fell against the banisters and it was just after that that I felt the lump.

I don't usually examine myself but about a month ago I fell and hurt my chest and when I was rubbing on a pain reliever I felt the lump.

The first patient clearly feels that there is some connection between her injury and the development of the cancer, whereas the second sees the injury as fortuitous, as it allowed her the opportunity of discovering the lump earlier. If the doctor ignores these narrative devices, the patient can be left confused and disorientated with many questions left unanswered. Alertness to the patient's story allows the doctor access to a deeper understanding of the patient beyond the purely scientific and pathological,[30] and for that reason it is every bit as relevant to diagnosis and treatment as scientific evidence.

2.4.4 Patient–patient anecdotes

As we have seen above, anecdote is often the way in which patients will relay to doctors the impact of their symptoms on their lives. But it is not just in the doctor's surgery where anecdotes are the means of lay communication on medical matters. Patients will share their own and their relatives' experience of illness and medical treatment through anecdote in the home, at work, and in the pub. These stories, it has been suggested by sociologists, may be one of the major means by which people decide whether or not they should visit the doctor with their problem.

A visit to the GP, or even more to the hospital clinic, is an important event, which in its turn will be conveyed by anecdote to family and friends. This is an important point for doctors to remember, as it is at this stage that the understanding, which the doctor thinks he or she has shared with the patient about their problem and its solution, may go awry. The story of the visit is told and the listeners will comment on it, drawing upon their own experience and knowledge, which is in turn often informed by anecdote. The scene might go something like this:

Patient: The doctor told me I had high blood pressure and I've to start taking these tablets.

Relative: Are you sure? I know Mr MacDonald down the road has got high blood pressure but he is twice the size of you and smokes like a chimney. He told me he had been getting terrible headaches and his doctor told him it was his blood pressure and he had to start cutting down on his smoking. Perhaps you should just try cutting down a bit too.

Patient: Yes. I don't feel unwell at all. I'll wait and see.

This kind of situation may contribute to compliance problems with some treatments.

Doctors must, therefore, be aware of the anecdote-sharing that goes on at home and in other contexts of patients' lives. Doctors need to be clear of what prompted them to consult, by asking patients for, and listening to, their account, and doctors then need to check on patients' understanding and compliance with any agreed treatment on subsequent visits.

2.4.5 Anecdotes as therapy

Allowing patients the chance to tell their story to its end can be an important part of the therapeutic process. This gives them the opportunity to order and clarify the experience of the illness in their own minds, and helps towards understanding it. It is surprising how difficult it is to listen properly to a patient's story to its conclusion; but it is important to do so because if the doctor interrupts, his comments are often completely ignored by the patient who wishes to finish his own narrative. As Peter Hoeg's heroine comments in his book *Miss Smilla's Feeling For Snow*:

Very few people know how to listen. Their haste pulls them out of the conversation, or they try internally to improve the situation, or they're preparing what their next speech will be when you shut up and it's their turn to take the stage.[31]

In summary, knowledge obtained through scientific endeavour in medicine is being vaunted as superior to knowledge obtained in other ways. However, learning from stories and anecdotes, and being alert to their use by patients, are essential to good medicine. This kind of knowledge enables us to deal with patients as an individuals and to respect their uniqueness as persons. As George Eliot in her novel *Middlemarch* said of Dr Lydgate:

He cared not only for 'cases', but for John and Elizabeth, especially Elizabeth.[32]

2.5 Interpretation

As we have seen, the diagnosis or prognosis relating to a specific patient derives from:

(1) evidence, properly so-called but based on the 'detective' model;

(2) information deriving from the patient's own stories or anecdotes.

Likewise, the doctor's recommended treatment derives from:

(1) evidence-based scientific research;

(2) anecdotes from other doctors in similar situations.

All this, however, must pass through the filter of the doctor's own judgement. In other words, it must be interpreted. But what is 'interpretation'? We wish in this section to consider what interpretation is, and how it contributes to clinical insight and judgement. We shall draw on some of the ideas found in hermeneutics.

2.5.1 What is 'interpretation'?

One of our commonest uses of the word is related to the expression, 'How do *you* interpret what he said, wrote, did?'. Here, the speaker is asking for the meaning that you (the observer) ascribe to what was said, written, or done. Inherent in the question is the implication that your interpretation might be different from mine or from anyone else's. The reason it is different is that your point of view or perspective on the subject might be different from mine or that of other people. An example might be if you are holidaying on a beach and see someone waving from the sea, you may well wave back, because your perspective on the situation is that everyone is on holiday and is behaving in a relaxed and friendly way. The life-guard who is scanning the sea for problems has a different point of view and may interpret the wave not as a friendly gesture but as a cry for help and rush in to rescue the bather. Gesture, then, is open to interpretation in different ways and that interpretation depends on the point of view of the observer, either in a literal sense—according to the position of the observer—or in a psychological sense—according to the feelings the observer has with regard to the situation.

This notion of point of view or perspective was introduced by one of the early writers in hermeneutics, Johann Martin Chladenius. Hermeneutics is the study of the interpretation of a text and Chladenius uses the ideas of hermeneutics in relation to historical method.[33] In the context of science, we might say that interpretations of phenomena can be correct or incorrect. Scientific enquiries focus on things that are not yet known but are assumed to be knowable, and knowledge of them depends on there being an appropriate experiment to uncover this. In order to frame such experiments, scientists will put forward interpretations of the phenomenon. These interpretations (as we have seen in Section 1.2.1) are called hypotheses, which will then, if possible, be subject to experiments to test their validity. The point, for the present argument, is that interpretations in this context may be correct or incorrect, but the answer is not known—and may never be known—by the interpreter. In order, then, for scientific interpretations to have some validity and for them to be taken seriously as possible explanations of phenomena, we depend on being able to say whether they are plausible or not. Nicolaus Copernicus, in postulating a Sun-centred system of astronomy in the sixteenth century, was not in a position to say whether his view was correct or not. He could say that this interpretation fitted the available facts better then the old Earth-centred idea, and was, therefore, a more plausible interpretation.

In some types of case, we can have situations where different interpretations of events or subjects can have equal *validity* and are not necessarily correct or incorrect. Politics gives many examples of this but literature and fine art may be the main areas where it is most commonly said that a number of different interpretations of a work may be equally plausible. One of the reasons that the plays of Shakespeare continue to fascinate theatre directors is that they can be played in many different ways. For instance, *Othello* can be seen as a play about a jealous husband, or about the trusting gullibility of the simple soldier, or about racial hatred. *The Merchant of Venice* can be played as a light comedy or as a comedy verging on tragedy, if the role of Shylock is given prominence by the director. We cannot say that any one of these readings of the plays is the correct one. They are all plausible as long as the text will support them. We cannot even appeal to authorial intention to support the most plausible reading, as Shakespeare does not stamp his presence on the plays. Artists may or may not chose to allow their own views of a work to surface. This may be particularly so of highly abstract art, where the artist paints something and leaves it to the viewer to make up his own mind about what the painting means.

This is not to say that anything goes in literature and art. Interpretations must be supported by a sensitive reading of the text, which will involve understanding of nuances and analogies employed by the author. The poem *Felix Randal* by Gerard Manley Hopkins contains this verse:

Sickness broke him. Impatient, he cursed at first, but mended
Being anointed and all; though a heavenlier heart began some
Months earlier, since I had our sweet reprieve and ransom
Tendered to him. Ah well, God rest him all road ever he offended! [34]

The poem can be seen as an account by Hopkins of this man Felix Randal, whom Hopkins ministered to as a priest in his last illness. But the poet's use of the Lancashire dialect in this verse brings Felix's voice to our ears and the poem becomes a vivid picture of this big, burly farrier at first railing against his illness and then accepting it with Northern fatalism. If our ears were not attuned to this dialect or if the style change was not pointed out to us, we would lose much of what was intended in the poem and our reading of it would be incorrect.

In summary, interpretations of things can be correct or incorrect, or more or less plausible; and it is possible to have a number of valid or plausible interpretations of the same thing. An individual's interpretation is guided by his own viewpoint. The correctness or plausibility of that interpretation will depend on how far that viewpoint is obscured by lack of knowledge or understanding of the subject.

Interpretation is, therefore, related to understanding. But what exactly is the relationship? There is no one conceptually correct answer to this. We can say either that interpretation is a process that *leads to* understanding, or we can say that interpretation *just is* understanding in a context of puzzlement.

An example of the idea of interpretation leading to understanding might be of the finding on an archaeological dig of a piece of carved flint lying amongst other such implements and animal remains. The archaeologist can see that the piece of flint has a blunt end and a broad sharp end, and its position implies that it might have been used in the process of cutting-up meat. He concludes that he has found a flint axe-head. This conclusion has come about entirely by interpretation of the shape of the implement, the position it was found on the dig, and by comparison with other such finds. The axe-head is then taken to a museum and is put on view as 'flint axe-head'. Does the viewer just understand that this is what the artefact is without going through any interpretative process? It may be that some interpretative activity is required by the viewer, as well, before he can conclude that this is an axe-head. That activity might be almost subconscious but it is necessary for the viewer to compare this object with axes as he knows them before he can see that this object is plausible as an axe.

As an example of the second idea of the relationship between interpretation and understanding, consider the situation in which we are not sure of the import of what someone is saying. In such a situation we engage in a process of interpretation. To confirm our interpretation we might ask, 'Do I understand you correctly...?'. In other words, interpretation just is understanding in the context of a certain sort of puzzlement. Indeed, another of the important originators of hermeneutics, Friedrich Schleiermacher, made no clear distinction between them and saw hermeneutics as the 'art of understanding'.[35]

From the point of view of this book, it is unimportant which line is taken. The important point is that interpretation is closely related to understanding, however that relationship is to be understood.

2.5.2 Interpretation and the clinic

Our account of the nature and scope of interpretation should make it possible to understand the central role it has in the clinic. Whether we are thinking of the diagnosis, prognosis, or treatment, it is clear that the doctor's decisions must be based on his interpretation of the evidence, including the patient's own anecdotes, as it relates to the individual case. That interpretation either constitutes or leads to his understanding of the case. It is our contention that interpretations are not in themselves in any sense evidence, but they are that without which evidence is blind and useless. It therefore follows that interpretation is a necessary component of clinical judgement. Before we can judge what the diagnosis is, or the treatment ought to be, we must have inter-preted the signs, symptoms, and anecdotes of the patient.

2.6 Knowledge and skills

So far in this chapter, we have been discussing how a doctor in a clinic might come to know what the diagnosis and treatment might be in an individual case, using the scientific evidence-base and the 'detective' individualized evidence-base, plus whatever can be gleaned and interpreted from anecdotes. This is all what a philosopher of medicine might call its epistemology or medicine's theory of knowledge. We have so far said nothing about the skills of the clinic. A discussion of the skills of the clinic, in general terms at least, will be the concern of this section.

The central role given to acquiring skills can be seen in the 'aims and objectives' of courses in medical faculties. They stress that the outcomes of such courses must be such that the student will be able to *do* various things rather than *know* various facts (see Section 6.8). Indeed, 'transferable skills' has become the catch-phrase of educational theory more generally.

We have been maintaining (Chapter 1) that scientific under-standing is a matter of acquiring systematic knowledge *that* certain facts are the case and are related in certain ways. In other words, our claim is that, when we speak of understanding why something is the case, how a trick is done, what a person is saying, and so on, what these senses of 'understand' have in common is that they are all related to the 'knowing that' family. Of course, when we play a game, or understand language, we are not necessarily rehearsing facts in our head. 'Knowledge that' or understanding is most often 'dispositional', in the sense that we just display it without thinking. But it is still a display of systematic knowledge. The same is true of many 'skills' in medicine. What the medical student or junior doctor may need to rehearse in her head is done by the experienced without thought. But it is a display of underlying understanding.

There is however an element of 'know how' or skill that is not reducible to 'know that'. Tying a surgical knot, for example, or giving an injection to a baby, are what might be termed 'motor skills', and they are not reducible to 'knowledge that'. Even here, however, the judgement of when, how much, for how long, to exercise these motor skills, must be governed by the doctor's systematic understanding of the patient's problem.

Obviously many of these skills are those of diagnosis, prognosis, and medical and surgical treatment. But it is important to discuss a set of skills that are much stressed as essential to the medical 'genius'—communication skills.

2.7 Communication skills

The importance of 'communication skills' is commonly thought, in medical literature at least, to be a discovery of the period 1960–90. It was alleged, with some justification, that doctors were deficient in such skills, and that it is of great importance for patient care that doctors should acquire 'communication skills'. Indeed, the medical stress on communication skills is part of a wider concern found in management studies and politics. This emphasis has tended to eclipse the importance of *what* is being communicated. For example, apologists for an unprecedented defeat of a Conservative Government in 1997 tended to say, 'We just didn't get our message across!'—as if it were a failure in communication, rather than in policy, which led to the defeat. Nevertheless, communication skills are important in general, and specifically, in the clinic.

It is, however, a serious error to think that the importance of communication skills is a discovery of the period 1960–90. The importance of such skills was noted by Plato (*Gorgias*) and by Aristotle (*Rhetoric*), and by many other writers in the ancient world. The Greek and Roman writers called such skills 'rhetoric' and saw them as both dangerous and as having a vital place in the education of a public or professional occupation. The importance of rhetoric was again emphasized in the Scottish Enlightenment. The term 'rhetoric' has bad associations in contemporary discourse. But the same kinds of point can be made via an analysis of explaining.

Explaining may be characterized as an activity aimed at producing the conceptually fitting response: 'Now it is plain to me, now I can understand it'. We suggest that explaining should be seen as a form of teaching, that form of teaching which is concerned with creating understanding rather than merely with imparting information. We may expect, therefore, that, like teaching, explanations will vary in style according to variations in many factors, such as the knowledge, ability, and interest of the listener.

To have communications skills, then, is to have the capacity to make and to measure explanations to fit the needs of the patient. The fault of the doctor lacking such skills is the fault of someone who thinks that there is one correct explanation and that his job is simply to deliver it. But the doctor with such skills is like a skilled keyboard player creating variations on a simple bass line. The bass line is the ground of medical fact but the good doctor is able to make something of this in a way which, in the words of the Scottish Enlightenment thinker, George Campbell, enlightens the understanding, pleases the imagination, moves the passions, and influences the will of the patient.[36] The good or humane doctor is, therefore, like a creative artist in the exercise of communication skills. But the 'when' and 'how much' requires humane judgement.

We shall turn now to an examination of clinical skills. Is there anything creative or artistic in the exercise of these skills?

2.8 Clinical skills and the 'art' of medicine

All doctors need to be able to examine a patient clinically and, despite the increasing reliance on laboratory tests and sophisticated imaging techniques, these skills are still an important and defining aspect of the doctor as 'expert'. Like communication skills, clinical skills can be seen in one sense as a method of gathering information about the patient, but in another sense they are also a medium through which doctors may convey humanity and display artistry.

The crucial point about the exercise of clinical skills is that doctors are permitted access to any part of the patient's body for examination purposes. Moreover, it is assumed by patients that doctors will wish to examine them and it is widely believed that overt consent is not required, even for the most intimate of examinations. Clearly, this belief raises many ethical concerns, one of which has been the question of chaperones, but our present concern is with the nature of this activity—is it merely the exercise of a skill or is there an art involved?

First, from the patient's point of view the most important consideration is the gentleness with which an examination is carried out. If asked, most patients will have a view about their doctor's clinical examination skills and they will compare doctors on the basis of how rough or gentle their touch was. Gentleness may be regarded as part of the exercise of the skill of examination, as without it the doctor is unlikely to gain the co-operation of the patient, but it also displays consideration and concern for the patient which is part of the humane approach.

Second, following on from this, clinical examination is important in terms of the development of a relationship between doctor and patient. Trust may be required for the examination to happen in the first place but an examination carried out with consideration, skill, and sensitivity, builds trust more securely than verbal communication.

Third, we would argue that in the hands of some physicians, clinical examination can be regarded as an art akin to playing the piano. At the same time as being aware of the patient's responses to the examination, and going through his knowledge of diagnostic options in his head, the physician's hands must be acutely aware of the plasticity of the skin under his hands, whether it yields to pressure or resists it, and whether the underlying structures feel 'right' or abnormal. The doctor may never have examined this individual before and all bodies feel different, so each act of examination involves the interpretation of a new sensation of touching. Some doctors can do this and others not. This does not depend on the quality of their training but rather on their innate artistry.

Thus, in the clinic the doctor spends much of his time in the exercise of skills, mainly those of communication and clinical examination. The information derived from these activities is added to and interpreted through knowledge and information from a wide variety of sources to enable the doctor to reach a judgement about a diagnosis and treatment plan. However this can all go awry if the patient's views are not consulted in the process.

2.9 Consent

The doctor's best efforts at diagnosis and treatment may receive a conclusive block in the clinic if the patient refuses the recommended treatment. A patient is, therefore, fully entitled to refuse the best evidence-based medicine, and may accept (because of patient–patient anecdote) a second- or third-best treatment. It is, therefore, important to recognize that in the clinical setting, the onward march of evidence-based medicine may be halted by the patient's refusal. Let us examine the meanings of the term 'consent'.

2.9.1 Consent as 'agreeing to'

The weakest sense of 'consent' is 'agreeing to' or 'accepting'. If we take an analogy from consent in political philosophy, then a ruler like Elizabeth I of England ruled by consent, in that she was popular and the people accepted or agreed with her policies of war with the Spanish or persecution of the Catholics. But her *right* to act in this way did not depend on their agreement: if they had not agreed, then it would not have mattered. This is the weakest sense of consent. In medicine it might be illustrated in contexts in which the doctor says: 'I am proposing to do x and y' or, 'I have just done x or y. Is that okay?'. And the patient says weakly, 'Yes, thank you doctor'. This strand of the consent doctrine does not confer rights on the patient.

2.9.2 Consent as 'authorizing'

A strong sense of consent is 'authorizing'. A might authorize B to do x and y on his behalf. In this case, B's right to do x and y necessarily depends on A's authorization. B is delegated to do x and y and the main responsibility for the doing of x and y rests with A. For example, I might instruct or authorize my agent to bid for me in an auction. This is too strong a sense of consent to be assimilated into the main tradition in medical ethics. It has the serious disadvantage in medicine of undermining professional autonomy: the doctor may feel that what I authorize is futile, and in any case it is up to him to make the treatment decisions, although the patient can legitimately refuse treatment. We shall discuss this further under the heading of 'consumerism' (Section 3.6). In the present context, however, we should note that there is good reason for maintaining the asymmetry whereby the patient may legitimately refuse a treatment or authorize, as distinct from agree to, the positive giving of a treatment. The reason is that the doctor is the expert on the patient's *medical* good—hence, only the doctor can authorize treatment. But the patient is the expert on his own *total* good. In the light of this knowledge of an overall or total good, the patient is entitled to refuse treatment, which might well be in his narrower medical good.

2.9.3 Consent as 'shared decision-making'

A third sense of consent is 'shared decision-making'. Shared decision-making has two elements. First, patient preferences and values are discussed by the doctor in the light of the doctor's treatment proposals or they could be mentioned in advance in a document. This type of discussion is necessary but not sufficient for what we are calling joint or shared decision-making. The second necessary condition is that this discussion results in the activating of a socially or often a legally sanctioned procedure. We can call this procedure the giving or refusing of permission.

These two conditions are together necessary and sufficient for this sense of consent. There are a number of important points to note about this form of consent. First, permission is given by both patient and doctor; each may permit the treatment or not. Second, 'permission' is a *normative* term. It is not like 'agreeing' or 'accepting', which are non-normative. I can accept a drink or agree to go to the cinema without any question of *rights*. But to give permission is to confer a right. Thus the patient gives or refuses the doctor a right to intervene, and the doctor gives the patient a right to have or not have the treatment in question. Third, the norms in question must be socially and, in the end, legally, sanctioned or legitimized by public policy. In other words, the parties must know and agree about procedures, and society more generally must know and agree.

Shared decision-making seems the most satisfactory model for consent in the clinic. The patient can be protected against paternalistic decisions deriving from doctors' or relatives' views of their total good. They can be protected because they can refuse permission through socially and/or legally sanctioned procedures. On the other hand, the doctor's professional autonomy is also respected in that he too is giving permission through socially sanctioned procedures. Moreover, responsibility is shared. In the first strand of the consent doctrine—agreeing or accepting—the main responsibility remains with the doctor. In the second—authorizing—the main responsibility remains with the authorizer. But in the third , the responsibility is shared by patient, doctor, *and* by society, which has sanctioned the procedures through its public policy.

2.10 Clinical skills as an art

In Chapter 1, we attempted to spell out the commonplace that medicine is a science, although one that relies to a varying degree on judgement. In Chapter 2, we have attempted to spell out the parallel commonplace that medicine is an 'art', and relies in different respects on judgement. Both are true, although the former applies predominantly to the research or knowledge base of medicine, and the latter predominantly to the clinical encounter. In particular, it has emerged that medicine is an art in the following senses: it involves the weighing of evidence in individual cases, the interpretation of the patient's anecdotes, and other features of the consultation; the exercise of skills, including communication skills in a manner appropriate to the individual case, and leading to the obtaining of informed consent. The common thread in this, which justifies the use of the term 'art', is that there can be no rules to direct the doctor. Even 'guidelines', a fashionable idea of ruling bodies in medicine, require interpretation in individual cases. A good doctor is, therefore, like a good musician: both require a basic technique and both must apply that technique to suit the occasion. In other words, in the clinical situation judgement is again central.

It might be argued here that we have claimed more in Chapter 2 than we have so far established, and that this is brought out by the analogy with the good musician. The good musician, it might be said, does not simply apply a technique to suit an occasion. Perhaps a craftsman does that, but the true artist not only individualizes his performance but adds some feeling, some humanity to the performance. So far the account of the good doctor has not shown how this element enters clinical practice. We have shown how the good doctor in the clinic is a craftsman, or artisan, but in what respects is she an artist? How is the good doctor a humane doctor? In answering this question we shall be showing how the judgements of the good doctor are not only technical judgements but also humane judgements. In other words, we shall complete the analysis of good clinical judgement by adding the analysis of 'humane judgement' to that of 'scientific judgement'.

2.11 Conclusions

1. Clinical consultation and practice is not simply a matter of applying scientific evidence to individual patients.

2. Scientific evidence provides a broad base for practice but evidence must also be individualized on the detective model.

3. Anecdotes are also a useful source of information on diagnosis and treatment.

4. Evidence and anecdote must be interpreted.

5. Clinical skills are an expression of the knowledge or evidence of medicine.

6. Communication skills can be seen as a kind of 'tailor-made' explanation.

7. The exercise of all clinical skills must be regulated by the patient's informed consent.

8. In the clinic the doctor practices the 'craft' of medicine, which becomes an 'art' when the element of the 'humane' is added.

References

1. Byrne PS, Long BFL, *Doctors Talking to Patients*. London: HMSO, 1976.
2. Balint M, *The Doctor, his Patient and the Illness*. London: Tavistock Publications, 1957.
3. Neighbour R, *The Inner Consultation*. Lancaster: MTP Press, 1987.
4. Pendleton D, Scofield T, Tate P, Havelock P, *The Consultation: an Approach to Learning and Teaching*. Oxford: Oxford University Press, 1987.
5. Sullivan FM, Macnaughton RJ, Evidence in consultations: interpreted and individualized. *Lancet* 1996; 348: 941–3.
6. Macnaughton RJ, Anecdotes and Empiricism. *BJGP* 1995; 45: 571-2.
7. Beard K, Bulpitt L, Macie-Taylor H, O'Malley K, Sever P, Webb S, Management of Elderly Patients with Hypertension. *BMJ* 1992; 304: 412–6.
8. Black JM, Norman GR, Kinsey E, Smith M, Report card from McMaster: student evaluation at a problem-based medical school. *Lancet* 1995; 345: 899–902.
9. Pendleton D, Professional development in general practice: problems, puzzles and paradigms. *BJGP* 1995; 45: 377–81.
10. Pickup AJ, Mee LJ, Hedley AJ, The general practitioner in continuing education. *Journal of the Royal College of General Practitioners* 1983; 33: 486–90.
11. Sackett DL, Haynes RB, Guyatt GH, Tugwell P, *Clinical Epidemiology*. New York: Little Brown, 1991.
12. Schmidt HG, Norman GR, Boshuizen HPA, A cognitive perspective on medial expertise: theory and implications. *Academic Medicine* 1990; 65: 611–21.
13. Department of Health, *New Advice on Oral Contraception*. London: HM Stationery Office, 1995.
14. Charlton B, Medical practice and the double-blind randomized controlled trial. *BJGP* 1991; 41: 355–56.
15. Hope T, Evidence based medicine and ethics. *Journal of Medical Ethics* 1995; 21: 259–60.
16. Macnaughton RJ, Evidence and clinical judgement. *Journal of Evaluation in Clinical Practice,* 1998; 4: 89–92.
17. Montgomery Hunter K, *Doctors' Stories: the Narrative Structure of Medical Knowledge*. Princeton: Princeton University Press, 1991, p.45.
18. Aristotle, *The Nicomachean Ethics*. Trans. D Ross. Oxford: Oxford University Press, 1980, 1140a20.
19. Plato, *Republic*. Trans. D Lee. Harmondsworth: Penguin, 1983, 332c.
20. Aristotle, op. cit., 1140b6.
21. Charlton B, 1991, op. cit.
22. A shorter version of this section appears in *Narrative-based Medicine* (ed. Greenhalgh P, Hurwitz B). London, BMJ Books, 1998, pp.202–11.
23. *The Times*, October 4, 1997, p25.
24. O'Donnell M, Trial by anecdote. *BMJ* 1991; 302: 56–7.
25. Brody H, *Stories of Sickness*. New Haven and London: Yale University Press, 1987.
26. Montgomery Hunter K, op. cit., pp.69–82.
27. Montgomery Hunter K, op. cit., p.74.
28. Gille A, The James Mackenzie Lecture: James Mackenzie and General Practice today. *Practitioner* 1962; 188: 94–107.

29. Mann RD, Breast implants: the tyranny of the anecdote. *Journal of Clinical Epidemiology* 1995; 48: 504–6.
30. Downie RS, Literature and medicine. *Journal of Medical Ethics* 1991; 17: 93–6, 98.
31. Hoeg P, *Miss Smilla's Feeling for Snow*. London: Flamingo, 1994. pp.36–7.
32. Eliot G, *Middlemarch*. London: Blackwood, 1871, p.105.
33. Mueller-Vollmer K (ed.) *The Hermeneutics Reader*. Oxford: Basil Blackwell Ltd., 1985, p.7.
34. Hopkins GM, Felix Randal. In *Poems by Gerard Manley Hopkins* (ed. MacKenzie NH). London: The Folio Society, 1974, p.92.
35. Mueller-Vollmer, op. cit., p. 12.
36. Campbell G, The philosophy of rhetoric (1808). Collected in *The Scottish Enlightenment: an Anthology*. (ed. Broadie A). Edinburgh, Cannongate Classics, 1997, p. 692.

3 Humane judgement

3.1 Medicine as a profession

The doctor–patient relationship is commonly seen as the central feature of medical practice: it is by means of this relationship that a doctor exercises professional skills and pursues the aims of medicine. The analysis of this relationship is the main concern of this section, since it is the key to the idea of humane judgement. It will emerge that, in addition to the need for the doctor to interpret and show insight into the symptoms and words of the patient—which are necessary also for the technical aspects of judgement—the humane doctor has ethical sensitivity and a broad educated perspective. The analysis of these factors will begin in this chapter and be completed in Chapter 6.

It must first be noted that the doctor–patient relationship is a professional relationship. What does that mean? The problem of defining, or even of roughly characterizing, a profession seems at first to be discouraging. Take first the large range of contexts in which the word 'profession' and its derivatives are to be found. We speak of a professional musician or footballer (as distinct from amateurs); we speak of a professional job as (distinct from one not so well done). These are distinct senses, since an amateur musician or footballer may well be a better player (and, there-fore, more 'professional') than some professionals (or those who earn fees from their activities). It might be said that we can step round the first problem by regarding these senses as derivative from the central sense in which, say, law is a profession. Thus, a professional musician earns his living by using his skills, as a lawyer does, and a professional job is one which shows a certain standard of achievement as (it is hoped) a lawyer does. To gen-eralize, we might say that a profession is a full-tine occupation by which a person might earn his or her living, and which is characterized by a body of knowledge and skills.

But this, while true, does not take us very far. Many occupations, such as being a farmer or printer, satisfy these criteria,
but are not normally considered to be professions. This suggests
that a better approach might be to consider the occupations that
call themselves 'professions' and discover what they might have
in common. Most people begin such a list of occupations with
law and medicine. Some may also include in their initial list
clergymen or priests, but, for reasons to be explained later, they
are not typical examples. More recently, accountancy, nursing,
teaching, social work, advertising, estate agency, and others have
been added. Are all these occupations and others to be included,
and if so what are the criteria for entry?

The hope here is that we can hit on a set of conditions, such
that all members of a class must have them, and if something has
such characteristics, it must be a member. But the trouble with
this search for definitions, in the form of necessary and sufficient
conditions, is that we are likely to have borderline cases. For
example, estate agency may have some but not all of the
characteristics of medicine. Is it to be included in the list of
professions or not?

One solution to this problem is to follow the method we took
in Chapter 1 when characterizing science, and drop the idea of
definitions as a set of necessary and sufficient conditions, and to
think instead of 'family resemblances' or overlapping characteristics. These will be the characteristics that will be most helpful
in the analysis of a dynamic and developing concept. New areas
of knowledge are opening up and bringing with them new
possibilities of public service. There will, therefore, always be
new contenders for the status of a profession. In case this is
considered to be a recent development, we must remember that
while surgery is nowadays considered as the paradigm of a
profession, it was not always thought to be so. The contemporary surgeon may well choose to forget his barber-shop
origins, but it was from such non-professional origins that
the profession has emerged. The concept of a profession is,
therefore, not static; so if we are searching for definitions, it
must be the looser idea of family resemblances that should be
our objective, rather than the stricter idea of a set of necessary
and sufficient conditions.

There is, however, a second and more serious problem attached to the search for the defining characteristics of a profession. Let us say that it is possible to find either a set of necessary and sufficient conditions or, more modestly, of family resemblances in terms of which most professional occupations can be identified. It does not follow that these criteria will be *relevant* for our purposes. For example, let us say that to be a profession, an occupation must satisfy the following criteria:

(1) it must involve at least 5 years training;

(2) it must have an appointed body supervising entry qualifications, negotiating pay and conditions of service for its members, and imposing discipline;

(3) it must have a code of ethics;

(4) it must have an annual conference.

Now it may well be that many or all professions satisfy these conditions. Let us further suppose that these criteria exclude the occupations that, for whatever reason, we do not wish to regard as real professions. Are these the *kind* of criteria we are looking for?

They are perhaps the kind of criteria we are looking for if we are engaged in a sociological investigation of some of the characteristics that professions at this moment in fact display. But criteria of this kind do not tell us what is important about a profession, or why professionalism should be encouraged or cherished in society. For this we require an approach that is philosophical or evaluative. What are the characteristics of a profession that are important to society? The answer to this will provide the clue to the idea of the humane doctor.

3.2 The knowledge base

The first characteristic that gives a profession social importance is its knowledge base. This does not mean that a profession is based exclusively on one discipline—on the contrary, professions tend to be eclectic and draw from various disciplines. As we have seen, medicine draws from the natural sciences and the social sciences. This condition, a base of knowledge and resultant skills, is clearly no more than a necessary condition for being a profession, for there are many occupations that have a solid knowledge base but which are not professions. For example, a systems analyst, an airline pilot, a physiologist, a film director, and many others, have considerable knowledge and skills but their occupations are not professions. We have already discussed at some length the knowledge and skills of medicine that satisfy this criterion and will say no more here, except to repeat that the generalized knowledge of medical research must be individualized in the clinic. There is a humane dimension to the process of individualization, which this chapter will explore.

3.3 Service through a relationship

A second characteristic of professions is that they provide a service for other persons. Now many professions, such as those involved in transport or public health, provide a service, but in the professions the service is provided specifically via a *relationship* between the professional and his clients. What is here meant by a 'relationship'? The answer to this question will provide the analysis of the humane doctor.

We can use the word 'relationship' in two ways: to stand for the bond that links two or more people; or to stand for the attitudes, which people so linked, have to each other. As examples of the first kind of relationship we might mention kinship, marriage, business association, or teacher–pupil. As examples of the second kind we might mention fear, respect, envy, contempt, etc. Thus someone seeing an adult with a child might ask, 'What is the relationship between that pair?', and receive an answer in terms of the first kind of relationship: 'teacher and pupil', 'father and son', etc. Or he might ask, 'What sort of relationship do Jones and his son have?', and receive an answer in terms of the second kind of relationship: 'Jones has a great affection for his son but his son has nothing but contempt for him'. Let us begin by examining the bond.

3.3.1 The bond

Typically in all professional relationships there is inequality of power. It can be argued that because of the dominant position doctors occupy in the relationship with their patients and because, as doctors, they must supply a service and often assess its success as well, they must be governed more than average by principles of ethics. In particular, in this context they must be governed by a desire to be of assistance to their patients, often called 'beneficence'. The ethics are formalized in a special 'bond', which usually takes the form of an institutional role relationship. The need for a formal bond is evident if we consider the significant interventions which doctors can make in the lives of their patients. We could approach this point in another way. We can characterize the doctor as someone who necessarily aims at health. It follows that the doctor's activities intimately bear on human good and harm, and therefore the state will take an interest in them. For example, the state will lay down broad conditions for the qualifications of doctors, or specify when a patient has a legal right to medical care, to hospitalization, and so on. There may even be cases, perhaps of certain infectious or psychiatric disorders, where the doctor has a duty to commit the patient to care against her wishes. In the latter case, the authority by which a person may be compulsory detained in a hospital, obtains legally in Britain from an Act of Parliament. The professional bond is constituted, additionally, by rather vaguer sets of rules, or even expectations, which doctors and patients have of each other. Doctors also refer to this as the 'ethics' of their profession, and the medical profession is very strict about enforcing its own discipline on these matters.

It is important that the doctor–patient relationship should be constituted, at least partly, by these legal and quasi-legal institutional bonds, for at least the following reasons. First, doctors and all health and welfare workers, by the nature of their jobs, intervene in existentially crucial ways in the lives of others. This is a serious matter and its consequences for a patient can be enormous. It is, therefore, in the interests of patients that there should be some sort of professional entitlement to intervene. In other words, if they are not simply to be busybodies, doctors must have the *right* to *intervene*, and if they have the right to intervene they must have duties and responsibilities; the concept of an institution encapsulates these ideas of rights, duties, and responsibilities.

A second reason is that doctors must ask about many intimate details of people's lives, for example, about their marriages; and they may also conduct examinations of people's bodies. Questioning of this sort, far less physical examination, can create situations in which people could be exploited or which could be embarrassing, even to doctors themselves. The fact that it is an institutional bond that brings doctors together with their patients, provides *emotional insulation* for both parties in such situations. Moreover, there must be some assurance that no untoward use be made of the information, that it will not be passed on to neighbours, etc. But the idea of an institution entails that of rules, and, third, the rules can impose *confidentiality* on the doctor and provide security for the patient.

Fourth, doctors are given a measure of *security* by virtue of the fact that they work inside an institutional framework. There are various aspects to this. For instance, it is good for all professionals to have ways and means whereby new skills and knowledge can be shared, and, in general, whereby members of a profession can support and encourage each other. Again, doctors require legal or similar professional protection from exploitation, unfair criticism, or legal action against them by their patients. Reciprocally, there must be some institutional mechanism whereby the professions criticize themselves and look for ways of improving their services to the public. These then are some of the reasons for which a complex legal and institutional structure has grown up governing directly and indirectly the relationships between doctors and their patients.

There are various desirable and undesirable aspects to this. For present purposes the relevant point is that when the doctor or other health worker appears to be acting as an individual, she is also acting as a *representative* of her profession and, to a lesser extent, also of the state. In other words, the individual action of a doctor or other health worker expresses also the collective values of her profession; individual responsibility becomes collective responsibility, since it is through individuals that their professions are represented. We might say that individual doctors represent their professions in two senses. First, they are the ascriptive representatives, in that the profession authorizes their actions, having sanctioned their training. Second, they represent the values of the profession insofar as they act in terms of its ethics, and its ethics is all pervasive in the actions and attitudes of the individual doctor.

The aspects of the professional relationship that we have been discussing can be expressed through the concept of a social role, understood for this purpose as being a set of rights and duties to be analysed in terms of institutional concepts. When individuals have accepted a role they are authorized to act in certain ways. This, the traditional view of the doctor–patient relationship, depicts it as a role relationship with the features we have noted; it is through the role so described that doctors and patients are bonded.

We have so far used the concept of a role as a way of linking medicine as an institution with the interests of *specific* patients, but it also enables us to refer to a broader social function that involves the doctor's duty to speak on matters of social justice and social utility. For example, doctors have a duty to speak out on broad issues of health and they might speak out against cigarette advertising. In this kind of way, the professions can be seen to have the important social function of regulators in the interest of general utility and justice. This is another aspect of the doctor–patient relationship, one in which doctors are concerned with categories or broad classes of patients, rather than with specific patients. We shall deal with this in more detail in Chapters 4 and 5.

In sum, then, the traditional view of the doctor–patient relationship depicts it in terms of a set of institutional bonds, legal and quasi-legal, which can be united in the concept of a social role.

3.3.2 Attitudes

To describe the doctor–patient relationship in terms of the institutional bonds that unite doctor to patient is to tell only half the story, and perhaps the less important half for an investigation of the 'humane' dimension in medicine. As we have said, relationships also involve attitudes, and it is to that aspect of the relationship that we now turn.

Notoriously, but perhaps not uncommonly, the object of the doctor's attitude will be the patient seen as a set of symptoms—

the fracture in bed three, or the neurotic who is always complaining, or the 20th patient who has come in complaining of feeling dizzy and sick. These ways of seeing patients will be perfectly familiar to most doctors, and no doubt there are many ways in which patients can be seen. When doctors see patients in such ways they are seeing the patient in terms of a range of medical sciences. The patient is being identified with a range of physical, psychological, or behavioural symptoms, and the understanding that doctors have of a patient seen in this way is technical.

Now received wisdom in medical ethics over the past few decades would condemn this way of seeing patients. We have been reminded by scores of writers that 'the patient is a person'. Yet it is surely essential that the patient should be seen as a set of symptoms if the doctor is to provide any effective treatment. There has been a huge volume of literature about 'deep caring' and the like, so that it is easy to forget that most patients are in the clinic for medical treatment and, therefore, must be seen in terms of their symptoms. But we can ask how, in addition to through the filter of their technical attitude, doctors can see their patients.

One answer might be that the doctor can see the patient as an individual. This does not mean discarding what might be termed the 'medical model' of the doctor–patient relationship, for to see patients as individuals may just be to see them in terms of their case histories. For example, a given patient, Mr X, might be seen as presenting with a *typical* set of problems—high blood pressure, high cholesterol, a smoker, and so on—and the doctor might see him in terms of *typical* biological and statistical probabilities as likely to have an myocardial infarction. But the doctor may *also* see him in terms of his individual case history, as someone who is anxious about his family, his job, and possible redundancy, who is working too hard, and so on. How does this individuating of the doctor's attitude—from seeing the patient as a set of generalized symptoms to seeing a patient who has *this* case history—change the doctor's attitude? The second attitude certainly adds something of importance, both medically and morally, but it is not clear that the *mode* of the attitude has changed. The doctor, as it were, is still on the outside of the relationship.

It might be suggested that what is missing is the element of the humane. Symptoms and case histories are for the doctor objective data, but for the patient they may well be a source of pain, discomfort, and anxiety. Additionally, the patient will be worried about what treatment, if any, the doctor can prescribe. In a word, what might be said to be lacking from the symptoms and the case-history models of the doctor–patient relationship is the awareness that the patient is *vulnerable*. We have already noted, in discussing the bond, that there is institutional and legal protection for patients because of their vulnerability, and it now seems reasonable to argue, that if the doctor sees the patient as vulnerable, the appropriate attitude towards this formal object is one of compassion or beneficence.

Something of importance has certainly now been noted. In particular, it has been recognized that the doctor must acknowledge the patient's humanity, and it is possible to do this through the adoption of the attitude of beneficence or compassion without losing any of the essential technical elements in the doctor's attitude already noted.

Nevertheless, there are two reasons why this suggestion falls short of a humane relationship. These reasons come, as it were, from opposite directions. The first is that a doctor may see a patient as vulnerable but not feel compassion, or anything at all. This does not mean that the doctor is emotionally stunted, but perhaps means only that he is very busy, or has found that feelings interfere with clinical skills and judgements. The second reason, which is perhaps the more fundamental, is that to see patients as vulnerable, suffering, or the like, is to see them in terms of only half of their humanity, and perhaps the less important half. Even vulnerable patients have a dignity in their suffering and this must be acknowledged as much as, or more than, their suffering. Indeed, when this dignity is ignored, we may find creeping back into the doctor's attitude elements of the paternalism for which doctors were much criticized a generation ago. Paternalism is a dangerous virus, and it is easily communicated via attitudes such as 'deep caring'. But even if the doctor can avoid falling into the trap of paternalism, there is still something missing in the beneficent attitude of the doctor towards the vulnerable patient, that is, if we wish to think of

the doctor–patient relationship as a form of a humane relationship.

It might be said that what is missing in this analysis is the
point that patients have *rights* to a doctor's services, and the
doctor's awareness of the patient's rights is the missing element
in the attitude as so far analysed.[1] But this suggestion must be
treated with great caution. If we really mean that the patient has
rights to *require* treatment from the doctor, we have transformed
the doctor–patient relationship into a salesperson–customer
relationship. Now there are a number of problems arising from
this approach, but for our present purposes it is not a helpful
move for the obvious reason that a salesperson and a customer
view each other as links in an impersonal chain. This model,
then, will not help us, even if we ignore the many problems
of seeing the professional doctor–patient relationship as a
commercial one. We shall discuss this issue in more detail in
Section 3.6.

It might be said, however, that to admit that patients have
rights, is not to be forced down the commercial road. The rights
that patients have may not require the doctor to deliver certain
services or treatments, but rather to have their views considered
and their consent or refusal of treatment respected. Concepts
such as 'patient autonomy' are in the background of this approach
and give rise to the 'partnership' or 'contractual' model of the
doctor–patient relationship. Let us consider briefly these slightly
different models.

The contractual model, as the term suggests, is based on a
legal analogy. It certainly limits paternalism, but it has serious
drawbacks for our purposes. First, a legal contract contains
specific undertakings, whereas a medical relationship tends to be
more open-ended. Second, the point of contracts is to remove the
need for trust between the contacting parties, but if trust is
withdrawn from the doctor–patient relationship, very little is
left of it. We have certainly not thereby created the humane
relationship.

The partnership model does better. Trust is essential to
partnership, and partnerships have a much wider remit than
contracts. Partnership suggests working together to plan, care,
and share responsibility for decisions. Above all it suggests the

mutual respect that is essential to a true relationship between persons. It therefore seems to be the model that opens the door to the humane relationship.

Unfortunately, it has some features that mean it does not fit all aspects of the doctor–patient relationship. A partnership presupposes that there are two or more autonomous persons respecting each other in a relationship of equality. But in the doctor–patient relationship, equality does not exist. The relationship is inevitably unequal in terms of its total power. The doctor knows more, and decides what to communicate to the patient and what to withhold. The patient is sick, vulnerable, perhaps in hospital or in a clinic, and as a result is insecure. Moreover, the doctor will have a team of other professionals to back up her decision. For these reasons and others, the doctor–patient relationship cannot be one of equality. It therefore cannot be a partnership in the full sense, although elements of partnership ought to be present. If, therefore, the humane relationship is one of equality, then the doctor–patient relationship cannot in principle be of that kind.

But the humane relationship is not necessarily one of equality; patients are vulnerable to the doctor's power. Yet, even if doctors and patients are not always in a relationship of equality, and even if through illness or serious disability a patient is not fully autonomous, it might still be possible for the doctor to see the patient in a humane way. Note too, in support of this approach, that the humane relationship need not be mutual; patients may be angry with, or distrustful of, their doctor. But, pulling together the threads, we might seem to be on the verge of a solution. We have argued that a patient can be seen as a set of symptoms, as a case history, as one who is vulnerable, and as one who has rights to be respected. It is tempting to say that to see the patient in a truly humane way is to see him in an organic unity of all these modes. If the doctor can hold all these together in a single attitude, she will have succeeded in seeing the patient in a truly humane way. Is the humane relationship the outcome of the doctor seeing the patient as an organic whole? Holistic care is certainly a fashionable term!

Unfortunately there is a serious drawback to this analysis. When we enter into a truly humane relationship with a person, it is to their being as a person that we are responding. But *patients* do not, in a comparable, way have a being. The concept of a patient is an abstraction from the totality of the person. In a similar way, we might enter into a humane relationship with Mr X, but not with a business man, even though Mr X is a business man.

Many philosophers would agree with this and argue that it is for exactly these reasons that patients should be seen as persons, because we can certainly enter into the humane relationship with persons. But what is here being proposed? Is it that the *doctor–patient* relationship should be replaced by a *doctor–person* relationship? This is an absurd view. The doctor must deal with patients, or in other words, with persons in certain restricted aspects of their total existence. Medical practice would become impossible if doctors and patients saw each other as persons in the full sense. It is the role relationship—the bond we have earlier discussed—that is the essential condition of medical practice. Have we then ruled out the possibility of the doctor–patient relationship being a truly humane relationship? Is the best we can expect that the doctor should be technically competent, compassionate, and respect the patient's consent and refusal of treatment? Well, if that were the relationship, it would be a good one, but it would barely be a truly humane relationship. Is there more to be said?

We could say that, in *addition* to seeing the patient as a patient, the doctor could see the patient as a person. What does this mean? We must draw a distinction between a 'medical good', the promotion of which is the intrinsic aim of medicine, and the patient's 'total good', which will include the medical good but much else besides about which only the patient is aware. There is a tendency in any profession to read the whole of someone's personality in terms of the limited aspects that one may be professionally concerned with. For example, a university tutor may see a student entirely in terms of her performance in essays or discussions, whereas for the student this may be comparatively unimportant. Likewise, there is an inevitable tendency for a doctor to medicalize every aspect of life and to forget that a medical good is only one among a range of goods. Certainly doctors must concentrate on promoting the medical good of

their patients—that is the essence of their aim as a profession—
but they must see this medical good in a larger context.

Let us take an analogy. Imagine a musical child who plays the
Chopin D flat nocturne at a music competition. The adjudicator
says to the child: 'You have played the nocturne accurately and
have observed the phrasing and dynamics faithfully, but you
will play it much better when you have had three love affairs and
two disappointments'. The adjudicator means that, although the
nocturne was played well technically, and the performance was
even a musical one, it nevertheless lacked a human context, or it
was played from the outside, or the inner meaning was missing.
In a similar way, a doctor could treat a patient in a way that was
technically excellent, and the doctor might also show compassion
and respect the patient's autonomous decision. Yet there might
be something lacking, although not anything the patient has a
right to complain about and, indeed, the patient might not detect
its absence. What might be lacking is the doctor's awareness of
the total context of the patient, the awareness that the patient has
a wider life. How can this awareness be shown? It can be shown
in quite simple ways, such as through a comment on matters
unconnected with the patient's illness—a football match or a book
the patient happens to be reading. Such incidental comments can
show an awareness that the patient has a *history*, a before and
after beyond the medical relationship, and a *geography*, places
and areas of life which have nothing to do with the clinic.

We shall look at three further questions: theoretical, ethical,
and educational. The theoretical question concerns the nature of
the attitudes involved. We said that attitudes are intentional—
directed towards formal objects. We have also said that, to the
extent that the doctor sees the patient as a patient, and he
logically must do that, the attitude will be a technical attitude or
range of attitudes, even if this technical attitude is also governed
by ethical principles, and so on. But we have also mentioned that
the doctor may also, at times, have a humane attitude to the
person who is, among other things, a patient. How is it possible
for the doctor to switch modes from one sort of relationship to
another and back? There seems to be a problem here if we
become fascinated by a misleading analogy. It is easy to think of
the intentional attitude as being like a searchlight, either on or

off. But perhaps (to continue the lighting metaphor) it is more like the flickering and varied coloured lights of a disco. It is possible for human beings to switch among a range of different technical attitudes, and then to a range of personal attitudes. It is this facility that makes it possible for the doctor–patient relationship to be at the same time both technical and humane.

The ethical point is that not all patients will chose to have in any sense, or at all, a humane or personal relationship with a doctor. They may wish to keep their personal lives entirely to themselves. This is their right and there is no personal failing on the patients' part if they should wish to exercise it. Patients, even terminal patients, may not wish to reveal themselves to anyone in the health-care professions. And they should be spared the attentions of the whole tribe of counsellors and pseudo 'experts' in emotional care. There are no experts in the exercise of humanity.

The educational point concerns the question of raising the consciousness of medical students and doctors to the possibility of these wider issues. Medical training is long: medical students tend to be taught together, without being much in contact with other students; doctors' friends tend to be other doctors. It is not surprising then that life for doctors becomes exclusively medicalized. Over the past two decades an attempt has been made to broaden the attitudes of medical students by teaching medical ethics. Now this discipline may help with decision-making, but to the extent that it is *medical* ethics it does not help with consciousness-raising. How, if at all, can the latter be done? We raise this question here for the sake of completeness, but will defer the answer to Chapter 6.

3.4 The humane attitude

We have argued that medicine is a profession and that a profession has two important characteristics. (It may have others, which we do not discuss here.) These are that it has a knowledge-base (discussed in Chapters 1 and 2) and offers a service through a special relationship. This relationship is constituted partly by formal bonds—legal and ethical—and partly by an attitude. In the case of a doctor we characterize this as a humane attitude. In describing the humane attitude we have tried to steer a course between two rocks. The first is the more dangerous. This one has painted on it clichés such as 'the patient is a person'. To be wrecked on this rock is to be killed with kindness, with totally unrealistic attempts at deep caring. Patients must remain patients or they cannot be treated. To have a humane attitude is to realize that the patient's medical good is only part of their total good. Humanity requires a broad-educated perspective. We shall deal with this in more detail in Chapter 6.

The second rock is less dangerous, but harder to see. This rock has painted on it the single word 'ethics'. If the doctor thinks that there is no more to having a humane attitude than to act on the principles of medical ethics, then she will hit this rock. Of course, an ethical sensitivity is important and, in particular, it is not only ethically but legally required to respect the competent patient's refusal of treatment, as we have already argued (Section 2.9). But there has become a tendency over the past decade for every non-scientific problem in medicine to be seen as an ethical problem. And, indeed, a tendency for ethical problems to be discussed in terms of principles of such abstraction that they are vacuous. This has been a consequence of the not wholly helpful influence of philosophy on the discussion of medical ethics. We claim that the doctor's humanity is wider than medical ethics, because there is more to a total perspective on life than medicine. We shall discuss what more there is, and how it can be taught, in Chapter 6.

Even if we avoid the dangers of too much sentimentality or too much medical ethics we must face up to the threat of two other dangers to the humane attitude. One is a threat—not a new one—from within the profession of medicine, and the other comes from outside medicine and represents a cultural change. The first of these we shall call 'medical affectation' and the second we shall call 'consumerism'.

3.5 Medical affectation

There is a danger to which any doctor writing about the nature of medical practice may succumb, and that is offering an elevated account of it, which is easy for outsiders to ridicule. One manifestation of this affectation, which is currently apparent, is the obsession with 'core values' that has gripped medical schools. The matter is sufficiently a threat to a truly humane attitude to be worth examining in some detail.[2] The problem has arisen because doctors have recently been grappling with their changing role in society. To this end, the first summit meeting of the profession since 1961[3] was held in November 1993, and its consultation document *Core Values for the Medical Profession in the 21st Century*[4] was produced. This document is sufficiently important to merit considerable reflection and comment.

In addressing the issue of core values, doctors have been responding to influences inside and outside the profession. Within the profession there has been evidence of low morale, dissatisfaction with work, and fear of litigation. This has largely been brought about by political and social changes outside medicine. The idealism that still exists in the profession has been undermined by consumerism (see Section 3.6). In addition, after almost 50 years of 'free' health care, patients' expectations have risen and high-quality health care is now seen as a right[5] not as something to be accepted with gratitude.

The profession has responded to these forces recently in three main ways. First, it has begun a radical rethink of the education of future doctors[6] and some hitherto fiercely conservative medical curricula are being swept aside in favour of a new structure incorporating problem-based learning theory and self-directed study.[7] (We shall discuss this in Chapter 6.) Second, doctors have begun to look more carefully at what they actually do, how well they do it, and at the evidence for doing it, and clinical governance and evidence-based medicine[8] are becoming the buzz ideas of the time. Third, there has been an attempt to look more philosophically at what being a doctor means in today's society and at what the profession stands for. It was this third area that the summit was convened to address, although any convincing answer to it would have to incorporate a consideration of issues one and two.

The main weakness in the document stems from the question that the conference set itself: 'What are the core *values* for the medical profession in the twenty-first century?'. This has encouraged the production of a list of good activities and attributes that might be associated with the practice of medicine but are not inherent to it or the defining of it. A better question might have been, 'What is the good doctor good at?',[9] thus rooting the question firmly in what a doctor does. An example of the vagueness attached to the document's broad central question is the list of 'basic and ancient virtues', which are given as 'commitment, caring, compassion, integrity, competence, spirit of enquiry, confidentiality, responsibility, and advocacy'. These read like a list of good things that, we might hope, would be associated with any upright citizen of the land, not just a member of the medical profession.

Indeed, there is another serious disadvantage attached to the document's moralistic use of terms such as 'virtues' and 'values'. These terms (largely used in logically incorrect ways) give the impression of an attempt to retain the high moral ground, which, as we shall see, has been the basis for the damaging gap between doctors' and patients' expectations. The final list of eleven 'core values' suffers from the same fault as the 'ancient virtues': it is non-specific and moralistic. Startlingly absent, is any clear statement of exactly what a doctor's responsibility to his patients is. Any discussion of core values in medicine at the present time should surely start with the question of what this responsibility amounts to and what its boundaries are. The doctor cannot be all things to all men. The therapeutic relationship between doctor and patient involves responsibilities on both sides. The doctor cannot take the tablets or stop smoking for the patient, and if the patient decides not to carry out the doctor's advice it may be because he does not value health as highly as other priorities in his life. Doctors must accept this.

Why does the profession so readily adopt the moral high ground, and why, indeed, is it encouraged in this by the public? The answer is partly ethical and partly historical. Ethically, regard for the profession and its members has arisen out of the need for patients to look up to those who have such power over them in the form of medical knowledge and skill, and who also have their tacit approval to perform intimate examinations in the exercise of this skill. Historically, this aura surrounding medicine has its origins in the rising status of medicine in the nineteenth century.[10] Moreover, it has recently strengthened because doctors are very successful self-publicists. Medicine , it seems, now has an answer to all of life's problems. If you are unhappy, take prozac; if you are bereaved, go to your GP because he is now trained in bereavement counselling; if you want a baby at the age of sixty there is even a doctor who will help you with that. It is now common practice for a GP to be summoned on an emergency visit to help with some family crisis that has suddenly blown up and will just as suddenly blow down. This image is not just to do with what doctors know and do, as this is quickly superseded by new knowledge (it has been said that medical knowledge has a half-life of 5 years).[11] Clearly, patients require of their doctors that they treat illness but they now expect more. Doctors are seen as the responsible members of a community to whom people might go for marital advice, job references, or for the signing of passport photographs. They are expected, therefore, to be honest and trustworthy. Great doctors attract great 'lay' honours; presidents of the main medical colleges usually collect knighthoods. Conversely, if a doctor behaves badly in his personal life, the public can be very censorious;[12] 'bad' doctors are seen as in some way destabilizing society and the public will come down very hard on them.

Do doctors want to perpetuate this situation? If so, it will mean an ever-increasing extension of the role of medicine, such that eventually it will become so diffuse as to be almost meaningless. In terms of medical education, the current hope is to reduce the number of different areas of study a student has to master. But if we are to contemplate an extended role for medicine there would need to be room, in effect, to squeeze in a social-work course, not to mention the mastery of alternative medical therapies. It seems more realistic for doctors to stick to practising medicine. To stress the importance of developing the idea of evidence-based medicine, is quite compatible with simultaneously stressing that medicine should be practised in a humane and compassionate manner. Being humane and compassionate, indeed having the 'basic and ancient virtues', may govern the *manner* of medical practice, but the *content* must rest on the bedrock of evidence-based medicine.

Of course, the profession has only deduced from patients' demands that they might wish an extended role from their doctors; we have not really asked them what they think. The 'Core Values' summit missed a great opportunity by not consulting the public for their views. It may be that the document was designed to stimulate debate inside and outside the profession, but with such a navel-gazing start this is extremely unlikely. In view of the fact that the stimulus for the debate came largely from the changing relationship between doctors and patients, the latter should have been included at the defining stage. In addition, it seems incredible that nurses and other members of the health-care team were not invited to contribute. Nurses, in particular, often have a clearer view of what it is that patients have found wanting in their doctors and their contribution is essential.

The sad truth is that while the medical profession still has a respected place in society, and many doctors wish to give it an extended role, medicine is not a panacea. Paradoxically, it is the respect that the profession enjoys, and the fanning of patients' expectations through the Patients' Charter, which is now leading to an erosion of its position. For medicine will not always work. Medicine is magic when it comes to transplanting hearts, treating diabetes, or even controlling blood pressure and reducing the risk of stroke. But when it comes to helping with the problems of daily living, doctors are no better than the next person and they have no greater expertise. Patients will come down hard on doctors when the magic is seen to fail, especially if patients are expected to defer to the purveyor of that magic as someone who represents trustworthiness, integrity, and stability in their world. It is this gap between expectation and reality that the 'Core Values' document should have addressed. That it failed to do so is one of the reasons it did not succeed in galvanising the profession.

If the profession continues to search within itself for definition it will fail. Certainly, the stimulus for debate on this issue has come partly from doctors who have held themselves up to be a kind of 'Everyman' doctor—a paragon of all the virtues, medical and personal. But just as important are the expectations of patients who have responded in the past to doctors' overweening self-publicity by expecting more and more perfect health care. It is time that doctors stepped down from the pedestal and got together with patients and other health professionals to tell it the way it is: doctors can't please all of the people all of the time, and sometimes they will fail.

Finally, at the risk of lowering the high moral tone of the 'Core Values' document, it should be remembered that most doctors have (and ought to have) commitments to other things outside medicine like family[13] or even leisure activities. It should not be considered morally reprehensible if doctors as persons value these things as much, or even more, than their profession. Thus, while the ethical, and more generally the humane, aspects of medical practice are of the first importance, it is also important for doctors to keep a sense of proportion about themselves and their wider role in society. Other occupations, from plumbers to philosophers, have a role and they too have their own values and humanity.

3.6 Consumerism

The second major threat to the humane doctor, indeed to the whole idea of a profession, comes from outside the profession. It is a particularly insidious threat in that many doctors do not see the implications of it and open their doors to it because it seems enlightened and in the interests of both patients and doctors to do so. This Trojan horse that will overthrow the very idea of a profession takes the innocent form of the slogan, 'Respect the decisions of the autonomous patient' or in its more consumerist form, 'Respect the rights of the patient'. Such slogans are dangerous because they are ambiguous. In one interpretation, we have already accepted such slogans as expressing the ethical bottom-line of good practice—the autonomous patient has an absolute legal and ethical right to refuse treatment. This ethical and legal right can easily become confused with another very different right—the right to require the doctor to make available a specific treatment demanded by the patient. This latter is a consumerist right, which requires a framework of consumerist ethics quite different from professional ethics. Of course, some doctors and patients may prefer the ethics of consumerism to those of professionalism, but it is important to be clear on the implications of consumerism for professionalism. We shall examine the history of this ambiguity.[14]

The idea of 'autonomy', of persons as self-determining and self-governing beings, is first discussed with a proper understanding of what it means by Kant (1724–1804). He assumed that people are essentially rational, although our desires may at times blind us. Decisions that are made as a result of dominant or blinding desires, he called 'heteronomous'. They are not truly the desires of the self, for they are caused by the non-rational aspects of human nature.

The Kantian tradition of moral philosophy, as it affected medical ethics, was modified by the liberal tradition of J.S. Mill (1806–73). Briefly, Mill argued that we have a right to do whatever we want, unless it can be shown that we are harming others. The key difference between Kant's approach to autonomy and Mill's lies in the respective emphases given to rationality and preferences. For Kant, a decision is autonomous if it is rational (whether it expresses our preferences or not). For Mill, an autonomous decision does express our preference, and it is less important whether the decision is rational. These traditions have merged and what has come out is autonomy as the expression of informed preferences or consent to whatever we do or is done to us by others.

This fused Kantian–Millean conception of autonomy, as preference or as informed consent, is one that can be absorbed by what we term the 'main tradition'. No doubt the doctor–patient relationship always involved some sort of consultation and discussion, and we can read the more recent emphasis on autonomy, on obtaining informed consent for all medical decisions, as an extension of, and an insistence on, that process of consultation. It can be seen as an antidote to the paternalism that was the pathology of the doctor–patient relationship in the past, and as a way of modernizing the relationship, of modifying it in terms of the modern ethos of openness in human relationships. It is important to note, however, that autonomous choice or informed consent in this sense takes place within the context of a professional consultation, with the patient retaining the right of veto to unwanted treatment, and the doctor retaining the right of veto to treatment professionally considered useless or harmful. But now let us look at the important difference when preference autonomy becomes consumer autonomy.

To set the scene, consider a genuine situation of consumer autonomy. Suppose that a person goes into a shoe shop and asks for a pair of shoes for walking along country lanes. He tries on various pairs, which do not appeal to him, and then his eye lights upon a pair of shiny patent leather shoes and he says he wants to buy them. A good salesperson will explain to him that they are not appropriate shoes for his purposes but, if he insists that these are the ones he wants, the salesperson has no duty to refuse the sale having advised against it; the customer here is exercising consumer autonomy. Can this idea be carried over into the medical context? Many ethicists think that it can, and, indeed, the British Government is encouraging the idea of consumer autonomy in health care to the extent that patients are being encouraged to see themselves as customers. The announcement in July 1999 that the Government is to set up a series of 'walk-in centres' is an example of this encouragement. The centres will be set up in supermarkets or railway stations specifically to answer what the Government sees as a consumer demand for more convenient health provision. Shoppers and commuters, there-fore, will be able to pop in for a quick consultation while they are visiting their supermarket or while they are waiting for a train. Let us examine the ethics literature on this.

Take the situation in which a patient, or relatives of the patient, request treatment that the doctor believes is useless or even harmful. In a study surveying the literature on this, Paris *et al.*[15] note that the doctors will almost always continue treatment if requested by patients or relatives, even if they regard it as futile. They do this because they believe that patient autonomy carries with it the right to whatever treatment the patient requests. Moreover, this view is supported by many US ethicists, who maintain that a physician is obliged to supply requested treatment, even if the request deviates from estab-lished standards or is, in terms of the doctor's judgement, in-appropriate.

In discussion of this we should note, first, that ethicists who hold this view of patient autonomy are surely mistaken, if they think that it follows from any interpretation of the doctrine of autonomy that people should be given something simply on the grounds that they demand it.

Second, we must remember that the principle of respect for autonomy applies not only to the patient but to the doctor, and if in the doctor's professional opinion the requested treatment is 'grossly inappropriate', then the doctor has no duty to provide it; indeed she has a duty not to provide it. This position has in fact been supported in the UK by the Court of Appeal. In a case in which a physician had indicated that he would not concur with a family's request to give a dying patient ventilatory treatment, if that became necessary to sustain the patient's life, Lord Justice Donaldson stated that:

...courts should not require a medical practitioner... to adopt a course of treatment which in the *bona fide* clinical judgement of the practitioner was contraindicated.

Lord Justice Balcome went further and wrote that he:

...could conceive of no situation where it would be proper to order a doctor to treat a patient in a manner contrary to his or her clinical judgement.

In other words, the Court of Appeal is here supporting the professional autonomy of the doctor.[16]

Third, let us consider the change in ethos or culture that is leading to the consumer-view of autonomy, and the implications of the change for the main tradition of the doctor–patient relationship. It will be remembered that in a true consumer situation, the shoe salesperson having advised me against buying shoes that are 'grossly inappropriate' for my purposes, has no duty to refuse the sale if I insist on buying them. What are the implications of importing these consumer assumptions into the doctor–patient relationship?

The most obvious implication is that medicine will cease to be a profession and will become a service industry. If that happens, the ethics of medicine will completely change. Indeed, some might argue that the need for ethics of any kind will vanish because the discipline of the market will replace the need for ethics. But we prefer to say that traditional medical ethics (which have grown up to protect the vulnerable patient against exploitation) will be replaced by the ethics of consumerism. And this is indeed being encouraged by the British Government. Let us look briefly at the ethics of consumerism.

Consumer ethics tend to highlight the following concepts. Consumers must have *access* to the services or goods they require; they must have *choice* of the goods or services they require; and this will involve *competition* between suppliers and a fair balance in the market place between supplier and customer; consumers must have *adequate information* on the goods and services they require, and the information must be expressed in clear language; it must be possible for the customer to obtain *redress* in the event of poor services or goods; the products or services must be *safe and subject to regulation* to ensure safety.

A consumer ethic of this kind underlies the idea of the free market and it is certainly appropriate in some areas of life. The question is whether it is appropriate in health care. It has at least two important implications: health care becomes a commodity, like any other in the market; and the carers make up a service industry. It is not possible here to discuss the far-reaching implications of such a change in ethos or to evaluate it. We shall simply note two implications of it, one relevant to the concerns of this chapter and one that will be taken up and developed when we examine the idea of rationing in Chapter 5.

The implication relevant to this chapter concerns the impact of an ethic or a culture of consumerism on the concept of the humane doctor. The points can be brought out in an over-simplified but sharp way if we note that a humane shopkeeper is an absurd or comic idea. In saying this we are emphatically not suggesting that shopkeepers are necessarily avaricious or dishonest. Traders in any market are required by the law to be honest, and by ethics also to be polite and helpful. But they do not need to be humane, compassionate, beneficent, or caring. We might become suspicious if they were! But we expect that of doctors.

Second, and perhaps more importantly, we must consider where we (the general public) want the responsibility for a medical decision to rest. Of course, a good doctor, as we have argued, will talk things over and provide appropriate information to the patient. But the responsibility for treatment must remain with the doctor and the responsibility for refusal must remain with the patient. The situation is different in the market. The seller must provide us with information on the goods, and perhaps advice, but the responsibility for buying the product, as well as refusing it, remains with the buyer. *Caveat emptor!* The financial implications of this will emerge in Chapter 5 when we consider rationing.

In sum, there is a threat to the humane doctor, and to the idea of a profession, from the outside—from consumerism. As we have said, it can be argued that the word 'threat' is tendentious, for what is coming about is a cultural change and, perhaps, a desirable one. If it is desirable, then the idea of the humane doctor must be replaced by that of the doctor as a supplier of goods and services. We do not think the change is desirable and so we shall continue the analysis of the humane doctor.

3.7 Insight and humane clinical judgement

In consolidating this account of the humane doctor—the one who has the qualities necessary to adapt the evidence-base of medicine to the particular patient—we shall analyse the idea of 'insight' and claim that the humane doctor makes insightful judgements. It will be part of the task of Chapter 6 to consider how far the education of the doctor can cultivate the capacity for insightful judgements.

There are two main ways of looking at this concept. First, an insight may be thought of as a perception that comes to someone suddenly—'a flash of insight'—and leads to a deeper understanding of something. Second, insightfulness can be seen as a tendency in a person to be able to see under the surface of something to its deeper meaning. We wish to consider these two aspects of the concept in turn.

Most of us will at some time have experienced this sudden flash of insight when a problem we have perhaps been thinking over for a while suddenly becomes clear. These sudden leaps in understanding are not usually the product of hard, concentrated puzzling over the subject; they often occur when we do not expect them, as Beveridge writes:

These sudden, large progressions occur not uncommonly when one is not thinking of anything in particular, or even when one is mildly occupied with something different, and in these circumstances they are often startling.[17]

Koestler calls these progressions the 'eureka process',[18] after the story of Archimedes with his crown in the bath. Beveridge also quotes from the descriptions of scientists whose ground-breaking discoveries have flashed upon them at unexpected moments. The theory of evolutionary change came to A.R. Wallace as he lay ill with fever in 1858 and was rereading Malthus' *Principles of Population*. In this essay, Malthus described the checks on human population increase and mentioned that these checks tended to eliminate the least fit. Wallace's mind started to ponder over a similar situation in the animal world:

Vaguely thinking over the enormous and constant destruction this implied, it then occurred to me to ask the question, 'Why do some die and some live?' and the answer was clearly that on the whole the best fitted live....Then it suddenly flashed upon me that this self-acting process would improve the race...the fittest would survive. Then at once I seemed to see the whole effect of this.[19]

These examples suggest that this kind of insight is the product of a mind primed and prepared for understanding after a process of striving for an answer. The answer then comes in a sudden flash, often at a time when the mind is focusing on something else, and the flash is accompanied by a rush of emotional excitement at the discovery of new ideas. These accounts relate largely to the creative work of scientists discovering new truths about the world, but is this kind of insight applicable to a more everyday situation such as the discoveries of a school pupil?

If we consider the elements of this kind of insight—the mind primed to receive understanding, the sudden flash, and the excitement associated with grasping new knowledge—they are all present in the case of the school pupil. It may not be the case that all new understanding comes about in this way but a schoolchild may experience this if—in the same way as the scientist—he has grappled with the problem of understanding something for a while. Unlike the scientist, the pupil's flash of insight is not a creative one, in that the understanding it produces in him is not new understanding for others, just for him. The 'eureka process', therefore, can be seen as a subset of this kind of insight in that it is creative and leads to new knowledge. Let us turn now to 'insightfulness'.

By this we mean the tendency of a person to be able to perceive a deeper meaning under the surface of things. When we describe someone as 'insightful', we regard them as sensitive, perceptive, and alert to the unexpressed emotions behind what someone says. The insightful person has highly tuned antennae for the unstated and is alert to nuances of meaning that others might miss. Those who experience the kinds of insights we have just discussed may well be insightful in this sense, but not necessarily so. Most of us will at some time experience sudden clicks of understanding but not all of us will be perceptive in the way that brings instinctive knowledge of something or—more usually—someone. In the clinical situation, I would be insightful if I realized that the patient in front of me really wanted to talk about her concerns about her daughter's drug use rather than the back pain she has officially presented with.

Insight or insightfulness concerns the *process* of understanding and is not meant to suggest that what is understood is of a fundamental nature. Detectives can have insights about their cases and doctors can be insightful in their dealings with their patients, as in the above example. This does not mean that they come across fundamental truths about their cases or patients, just that they approach the evidence or person in front of them in a sensitive and perceptive way; and that they are alert for any clues, whether these come via their reason, senses, or instinct. Insightfulness is one reservoir that supplies sound judgement.

How does insight relate to understanding? In answering this question, it is helpful to recall the connection that exists between interpretation and understanding. In discussing that connection (Section 2.5.1), we maintained that we can say either that interpretation *leads to* understanding or *just is* understanding in a context of puzzlement. The same is true of insight. Insight, or the bringing together of two apparently unconnected thoughts or perceptions, can be seen as leading to understanding or as constituting one mode of it.

3.8 Humane judgement and the humane attitude

We have suggested that the concepts of interpretation and insight lead to, or constitute, understanding. It is not that there are two conceptual layers here: there is one conceptual layer, which is describable in different language in different contexts. It is this understanding that is the basis for humane judgement.

Ethical sensitivity is also involved in humane judgement, but in a different way. It *governs* judgement rather than constitutes its basis. But for simplicity, we shall regard all three as the components of humane judgement, which in turn is an expression of the attitude of the humane doctor (see diagrammatic summary p.xii).

It might be objected that we have too many conceptual layers here; that if we speak of humane judgement, we do not also need to speak of a humane attitude. This objection can be answered by drawing the distinction between a disposition and episodes in which it is expressed. For example, someone may have a courageous disposition and this will be shown in courageous actions. In a similar way, we wish to maintain that the humane attitude is shown in humane judgement. There are not really two different things here, but one thing described in different contexts.

3.9 Best evidence-based practice

We are now in a position to be able to sum up the next stage of our analysis of clinical judgement. We saw in Chapter 1 the importance of medical research and brought out that its evidence-base rested on a foundation of judgement. When this evidence-base is used in the clinic it has to be individualized, in the manner of a detective as he pursues a particular case. The judgements that derive from the research base and detective work we can call scientific or (more aptly) technical judgements. They are 'scientific' or 'technical' because they satisfy, to a greater or lesser extent, the criteria for well-founded evidence at either the generalizable (science) or the individual (detective-like) levels. But they are 'judgements' because they rely on the insights and interpretations of the clinician. We have offered an analysis of 'interpretation' (Section 2.5) and 'insight' (Section 3.7), which are the essential components of judgements of any sort.

In Chapter 3, we concentrated on the question of what it means for a doctor to be 'humane'. Important points here are that medicine is a profession and 'doctor' and 'patient' are role-words with the built-in impersonality that role-relationships necessarily have. We then argued that, granted its necessary formality, a doctor–patient relationship could also be humane (Section 3.4). The humane attitude shown in this relationship can be expressed in humane judgement. We shall later—in Chapter 6—complete our analysis of the humane attitude by adding the component of 'educatedness'. In the meantime, our provisional conclusion is that good clinical judgement, then, is a compound consisting of a fusion of technical judgement and humane judgement and, governed by ethical sensitivity, it will issue in best evidence-based practice.

3.10 Conclusions

1. The good doctor has scientific knowledge, communication skills, and 'humanity'.

2. The doctor's 'humanity' is wider than what is usually considered 'ethical', although the latter is included.

3. It is important that doctors do not exaggerate the importance of their role in society, and that they resist attempts to turn the doctor–patient relationship into a purely market or supplier-consumer relationship.

4. 'Insight' or 'being insightful' are complex ideas, which are none-the-less integral to the clinical situation.

5. Being insightful can be added to the ability to interpret, as forms of understanding, and components of the concept of judgement.

6. Scientific knowledge and skills, communication skills, ethical sensitivity, and a humane attitude, are all needed for the interpretative skills and insights of good clinical judgement.

7.	Clinical judgement is a unity, but its components are technical judgement and humane judgement.

References

1.	Randall F, Downie RS, *Palliative Care Ethics* (2nd edn). Oxford: Oxford University Press. 1999, pp.39–47.
2.	Macnaughton RJ, Core values: doctor or everyman? *BMJ* 1996; 313: 120–1.
3.	Smith R, Medicine's core values. *BMJ* 1994; 309: 1247–8.
4.	*Core Values for the Medical Profession in the 21st Century:* Report of conference held on 3/4 November 1994. London: BMA, 1995.
5.	*The Patients' Charter.* London: HMSO.
6.	General Medical Council. *Tomorrow's Doctors: Recommendations on Undergraduate Medical Education.* London: GMC, 1993.
7.	Glasgow University Faculty of Medicine: Proposals for a new undergraduate curriculum 1996 (unpublished).
8.	Davidoff F, Haynes B, Sackett D, Smith R, Evidence-based medicine. *BMJ* 1995; 310: 1085–6.
9.	Downie RS, Charlton B, *The Making of a Doctor.* Oxford: Oxford University Press, 1992.
10.	Youngston AJ, Medical education in the later 19th century: the science take-over. *Medical Education* 1989; 23: 480–91.
11.	McCormick JS, *The Doctor: Father Figure or Plumber.* London: Croom Helm, 1979.
12.	Top Tory Drugs Disgrace. Leader in *Pulse* 1995; 55: 1.
13.	Smith, op. cit. p.1247.
14.	Randall and Downie, op cit., pp.6–10.
15.	Paris JJ, Schreiber MD, Statter M, Arensman R, Siegler M, Sounding Board. *New England Journal of Medicine,* 1993; 329, (5): 354–7.
16.	Re J (a minor) (1992), 4 *All England Reports,* 614.
17.	Beveridge WIB, *The Art of Scientific Investigation.* London: William Heinemann Ltd., 1950, p.54.
18.	Koestler A, *Insight and Outlook: an Inquiry into the Common Foundations of Science, Art and Social Ethics.* London: Macmillan, 1949, p.254.
19.	Beveridge, op. cit., quoting AR Wallace, p.69.

4 Judgement in public health

4.1 Introduction

We have so far concentrated on the complex ways in which the evidence-base of medicine is modified by judgement in clinical practice. Thus, patient anecdotes and patient consent or refusal of given treatments affect the options available in a clinical situation. Moreover, the doctor's scientific attitude is modified by his ability to interpret and to have insights about the individual patient. But, as distinct from clinical practice, there is another domain of medicine with its own distinctive evidence-base and its own need for judgements of a different sort—this is the domain of public health medicine, formerly called 'community medicine'.

The domain of public health medicine is an important one. Indeed, it is widely recognized that the huge improvements in the health and longevity of Europeans and North Americans this century are much more due to improvements brought about by public health medicine than they are by clinical medicine. The contemporary emphasis on expensive, high-tech medicine has, in fact, affected the general health in only marginal ways. In discussing the evidence-base of public health medicine separately from that of clinical medicine, therefore, we are not to be taken as seeing it as an unimportant appendix to clinical medicine (although Government expenditure in the area seems to endorse the 'unimportant appendix' point of view); rather we are discussing it separately because of the different way in which the insights affect the evidence. We shall begin by considering the nature of public health medicine.

4.2 Public health medicine and its evidence-base

Let us begin by accepting the World Health Organisation (WHO) definition of the term 'public health',[1] used also in the UK in the Acheson report:

Public health is the science and art of preventing disease, prolonging life and promoting health through organized efforts of society.[2]

This definition suggests that evidence problems can arise in public health over preventing disease and promoting health. 'Prolonging life', if it is not achieved by preventing disease or promoting health, is a matter for clinical medicine and will not be discussed separately in this chapter. Issues may also arise over 'the organized efforts of society' and over what it means to say that public health is both a science and an art. We shall conduct our discussion, then, under these headings and try to encompass a representative selection of issues, including some with international implications.

But let us first examine the evidence-base of public health medicine. It will quickly emerge why policies based on that evidence rely more on interpretation and insight than do judgements in clinical practice. In particular, moral and political considerations are of the first importance in shaping the evidence on which public health medicine is based.

Public health medicine is based on the science of epidemiology, which many public health specialists see as the ultimate triumph of evidence-based medicine. But epidemiology is a difficult and uncertain discipline. It is thought to be justified in the public arena as a source of objective information for all those who have vested interests in outcomes and natural histories of diseases and their treatments. Yet the language of its science is neither easy to approach nor easy to understand, and its findings are couched often in terms that seem equivocal. Risks and benefits are qualified and couched in probabilistic terms. Nevertheless, these conclusions are to be used to define 'best practice', cost–benefit algorithms, 'right action', informed consent or choice, political choice and action, community health decisions, and even health advocacy programmes. The conclusions are drawn from numerical data, and gain their status from the status accorded to objective data.

Yet many of its practitioners are uneasy about the way that epidemiology is conceived, practised and used. In a mock indictment of the science, Shy has attempted to restate the mission of epidemiology:

By essentially assuming that risk factors for disease in individuals can be summed to understand the causes of disease in populations, academic epidemiology has limited itself to a narrow biomedical perspective, thereby committing the biomedical fallacy of inferring that disease in populations can be understood by studying risk factors for disease in individuals. Epidemiology should be redefined as a study of the distribution and societal determinants of the health of populations. This definition provided a stronger link to the primary mission of public health and places an appropriate emphasis on the social, economic, environmental and cultural determinants of population health.[3]

Like all components of the health endeavour, epidemiology is inescapably moral in all its purposes. Because it intends to guide health-care decisions at many levels, epidemiology shares the moral purpose of all health-related activity. It seeks to determine what it is best for health-care workers to do, where 'best' is in some way defined by societal values assigned to the primary good of health. By helping to determine 'best practice', epidemiology clearly asserts its vision of itself as one of the most important ways of bringing a computational dimension to the essential morality of public policy. Therein lies both its strength and its weakness, for it must, by its very nature, operate in an uneasy hinterland between the plains of objective evaluation and the poorly charted mountains of community values. This is the core of the problem to be examined in this chapter, the problem of assigning meaning to epidemiological studies. We shall examine the various ways in which the evidence-base of the sub-divisions of public health medicine (as defined by the WHO) are affected by the interpretations and insights, especially the moral and political judgements, of those using epidemiological studies.

Typically in epidemiology, numerical evidence and judgement make up a 'seamless garment'. For example, the following are a few of the phrases in which fact and judgement are married: 'burden of disease', 'poverty, homelessness, and poor housing conditions', 'violence', 'the figures show an improvement', 'protection against diphtheria is inadequate', 'there is also concern that...', 'vulnerable group', 'a mixture of good news and bad news'. Much epidemiological writing is indeed explicit that many of the lessons are ethical.[4] The point we wish to make, however, is not the obvious one that, granted the figures, we can make ethical judgements. Our point is that the very selection and compilation of these figures, as distinct from other figures, indicated a prior ethical judgement. The decision to carry out epidemiological studies in certain areas and to compare the figures compiled with other areas of the world, or with other historical periods, is itself an ethical decision. The 'evidence' is there because the ethical insight has first been there.

Epidemiologists are sometimes blinded to the evaluative nature of their discipline by their use of the term 'health inequality'. Epidemiological studies frequently blur the differences between equality or inequality on the one hand, and equity or inequity on the other. Let us examine this distinction in the context of public health.

The distinction can best be described by looking at those factors that can influence health and health care. It is possible to divide inequalities into those that are unavoidable, and hence where questions of equity do not arise, and those that might be avoided, and thus raise issues of equity. Let us look at some examples.[5] In discussing these examples, we must always remember that what is 'unavoidable' at one point in history becomes 'avoidable' at another.

First, natural or biological variations, such as age, sex, and race, and genetic background could be considered as factors that cannot be changed and thus, any inequalities related to them are unavoidable. For example, older men have a higher incidence of heart disease than younger men, a clear example of an inequality. But no one would consider this related to inequity, except to the extent that we have neglected risk factor reduction in the elderly.[6]

Secondly, lifestyle and behaviour, if freely chosen, can result in inequalities in health. As an example, cigarette smokers have a higher incidence of lung cancer than non-smokers. This is an inequality, but to the extent that it is created by choice, it is not inequitable. Indeed, selective uptake of health promotional initiatives, for example, by middle class groups, could even increase inequalities in health, but could not be considered as unfair, unless it could be established that health promotion is selectively targeted on these groups.

Third, lifestyle and behaviour, if not freely chosen, and which results in poor health, is likely to be considered as avoidable by society and thus unfair. A behaviour chosen through a lack of resources, housing conditions, overcrowding, dangerous working conditions, exposure to environmental hazards, or lack of adequate public health response, would be an example of this. Disabled people often suffer unfairness (inequity), which compounds their already unequal health.

Fourth, inadequate access to health care or other public services might be inequitable if the cause were avoidable. For example, financial considerations that resulted in a failure to use transport, might be one such factor. Another might be lack of access to information about services due to learning or language problems, or the information not being available. This lack, or inequity, could lead to inequalities of access because of the restriction of choice and opportunity.

In summary of this discussion of the principle of justice, we can say that these examples bring out that equity is about fairness and justice, and implies that everyone should have an opportunity to attain his or her full potential for health. Inequalities exist in health and health care. Some of these are unavoidable, and thus could not be considered unfair or inequitable. Others are avoidable. It is this latter group in which the inequalities are inequitable, to which further attention might be addressed.

But for the purposes of our argument, the point is that evidence and ethical judgement are intertwined in public health medicine, and the failure of epidemiologists to notice this can give rise to confusions of policy. There is, indeed, an aspect of public health medicine that makes its ethical base of the first importance. Let us examine this by comparing public health medicine with clinical medicine from the ethical standpoint.

4.3 Public health ethics and health care ethics

The clinician is typically in a one-to-one relationship with a patient who has requested an interview because of a felt problem. The clinical imperative is, therefore, that something must be done, including the giving of advice. The public health specialist, on the other hand, does not have a specific patient with whom he is in a special relationship, and has received no request from a patient.

It could be said that the public health specialist responds to a collective cry from individuals in a community, when some medical problem occurs that affects a large number of people in a locality. One example is the outbreak, in 1997, of *Escherichia coli* 0157 in Wishaw in central Scotland. But here, again, there is no continuing relationship between the specialist and the affected group of individuals, and, therefore, no opportunity for those individuals to express their views on the public health response.

The public health specialist therefore is:

(1) making a judgement about what it is in people's interest to have, whether they have requested it or not; and

(2) dealing with populations, groups or societies rather than individuals.

The ethical consequence of these features are that public health generates problems concerned with issues such as paternalism and individual rights, which are broadly (i.e. non-party) political in their implications, and therefore where judgement is of the essence. But the judgement should follow from the evidence. Thus for any specific intervention (legislation for clean water, a programme of immunization, restriction on smoking in public places, or whatever), the necessary precondition of implementation is that it will improve the health of the public—and this improvement must be objectively demonstrable.[7] According to this approach, effectiveness must be established by scientific means, such that all rational and competent judges can agree on the facts.[8] The most common technique for establishing effectiveness of this kind is through the discipline of epidemiology. But, as we have already seen, clear and certain conclusions may not always be obtainable.

The conclusion, then, is that judgements are of vital importance to public health medicine, both in that judgement is integrated with epidemiology, and in that social and political issues can affect the implementation of the conclusions of epidemiology. Let us now move on to another aspect of the WHO definition of public health medicine and consider 'prevention'.

4.4 Prevention

There is sometimes confusion between *prevention*, which is the abolition or reduction in the incidence of the disease; *avoidance*, which is keeping clear of risk factors; and *protection*, which may limit the spread of disease, say by vaccination or immunization. For example, public health policy may encourage the prevention of malaria by swamp-clearing programmes and thus aim at the elimination of the source of the disease; or travellers may avoid catching the disease by avoiding certain geographical areas; or they may be protected against it by being given tablets. All these practices are loosely called 'prevention'. Of course, the categories will sometimes overlap. For instance, immunization or vaccination programmes, which are really protection programmes, may lead to a reduction in the incidence of a disease, or even to its elimination, as in the case of smallpox. But this overlap does not always occur. The compulsory wearing of seatbelts is often regarded as a preventive measure. But it does not prevent accidents; only good driving and safer roads and vehicles do that. It gives a measure of protection against accidents.[9]

It might seem that there is no need to provide any ethical justification for prevention: it is self-evidently a good thing. While this may be true, the general public and governments do not always act as if it were so. From the point of view of government, it seems that much more money goes in the direction of health care than of prevention, and from the point of view of the public, there is often an attitude of scepticism towards many preventive measures, and even more towards what is now called 'health promotion'. Prevention as a general policy, therefore, requires some justification. There is an economic justification, that prevention is usually cheaper than care; medical justification, that some diseases are probably not completely curable, so their occurrence should be prevented; and an ethical justification, that prevention avoids the pain, misery, and grief of disease. It is also possible to include the economic and medical justifications in a wide sense of 'ethical justification'. As we shall see, however, this general ethical justification of prevention does not always apply to specific areas of prevention, and even when it does, there are those who argue that the benefits of prevention can be outweighed, in some cases, by the ethical costs. Let us look at some examples.

Take the fluoridation of local water supplies. From the 1930s it was noted that there was a correlation between levels of fluoride in the drinking water and levels of dental caries. This suggested a preventive policy of introducing fluoride where the level was low. There were objections, on the grounds of undesirable side-effects, such as Downs Syndrome and, more recently, cancer. But a Working Party in Britain[10] found no evidence for such claims, and other scientific groups have reached the same conclusion. The ethical objection remains, however, that adding fluoride to the water supply can count as compulsory medication and, as such, it is a violation of individual rights as laid down in the UN Declaration of Human Rights. Rights, of course, are not inalienable and can be overridden when the survival of the public requires it. But it is doubtful if the prevention of dental caries can count as a justification for ignoring rights. Note that there is really no solution to this dispute. One position or the other must be overruled.[11]

The issue of vaccination for rubella raises rather different issues. The vaccine for rubella works by providing a benefit to the children of those to whom it is given. Now the vaccine can be given to girls only, or to both girls and boys. If it is given to girls only, there is little effect on the transmission or eradication of the disease. A 'girls-only' policy is, therefore, a 'protection' rather than a 'prevention' measure. If, on the other hand, the vaccine is given to both girls and boys, and if the uptake is over 90%, we have a preventive measure that will eventually lead to the eradication of the disease. But if the second policy is followed and the uptake is low, say about 60%, then we have a situation that is harmful to the children of the unvaccinated young female population, for they will be much less likely to develop natural immunity. The ethical issues, then, are these. If we (the public) want the benefits of prevention, then we must also put up with a degree of compulsion to ensure a high uptake. If compulsion is ethically or politically unacceptable, then the best policy, to avoid harm, is to offer protection to those at risk. Again there is no ethically correct answer; a judgement must be made.[12]

4.4.1 Screening

Another public health activity that falls, in general terms, into the category of prevention, is that of screening. Screening can be defined in various ways, but a simple definition is provided by Stone and Stewart:[13]

Screening is a preventive activity which seeks to identify an unsuspected disease or pre-disease condition for which an effective intervention is available.

Screening is currently a fashionable medical activity. The demand for it is being encouraged by governments and by certain patients' organisations.

Politically, it seems desirable because there is a belief that prevention saves money, and successive governments have, therefore, set up various screening programmes. A national screening programme for cervical cancer was set up in the UK in 1964, and a programme for breast cancer was established in 1988 for women aged 50–64 years. The establishment of such programmes has been enthusiastically supported by various women's groups. Indeed, such is the current demand for screening that Shickle and Chadwick,[14] in a discussion of the ethics of screening, ask whether 'screeningitis' is an incurable disease. If it were, no doubt there would be demand for a screening programme!

It is possible to screen for many conditions, but screening programmes must satisfy ethical criteria. First, they must satisfy the informed consent criterion for any sort of medical intervention. Second, since screening initiatives tend to be profession-driven, rather than individual-driven, there is an additional responsibility for the professional to justify an intervention that may not have been requested. Third, some screening procedures carry health risks, and all of them are likely to be accompanied by discomfort, anxiety, and inconvenience for symptomless individuals. Fourth, any screening programme carries with it the risks of the false-positive or the false-negative. Thus screening requires as much ethical justification as other medical interventions. Moreover, since screening programmes can be expensive in the aggregate, they require evaluation. Once again, therefore, the ethical principles of justice and utility must be used in the justification of screening programmes.

4.5 Health promotion

The Acheson Report definition of public health makes it clear that public health medicine must not only prevent disease but promote health. The literature of the new public health, and especially health promotion, tends nowadays to have a complex view of the concept of health, and to distinguish various elements within it.

The first of these is often called 'negative health', or the absence of ill-health. Ill-health itself is a complex notion comprising disease, illness, handicap, injury, and other related ideas. These overlapping concepts can be linked if they are seen on the model of abnormal, unwanted, or incapacitating states of a biological system.

The second idea of 'positive health' has appeared more recently in published reports. The origins of this idea are in the definition of health to be found in the preamble to the Constitution of the WHO:

Health is a state of complete physical, mental and social well-being, and not merely the absence of disease or infirmity.[15]

It follows from this definition, that 'well-being' is an important ingredient in positive health.

A third idea in the concept of health is that of 'fitness'. Fitness in its most obvious sense refers to the state of someone's heart and lungs. To be fit in this sense is to have a place on a scale ranging from being able to climb stairs or run for a bus, without getting out of breath, to being able to run a marathon or climb Mount Everest. Fitness can also be used in a related but broader sense, which we might call the 'sociological' as opposed to the 'heart and lungs' sense. In the sociological sense of fitness, a person is fit *for* some occupation or job. This means that people have the necessary health to enable them to perform the job adequately without, for example, too many days off work.

The WHO definition refers to the 'mental and social', as well as to the physical. Nevertheless, the mental and social components of health are the poor relations of the health services and do not receive adequate attention. It is certainly true that mental health is most often taken to be the absence of mental ill-health. The idea of positive mental health or mental well-being is an obscure one, and perhaps it is ethically dangerous if it implies that eccentricity and single-mindedness are to be discouraged, and the balanced and conformist personality encouraged.

The idea of 'social well-being' is, in fact, just as obscure as that of mental well-being, although at first sight it does not seem to be a difficult notion. What does it mean? In one sense, 'social well-being' refers to the skills and other abilities that enable us to form friendships and relate to other people in conversation and through the many different sorts of contact, which are part of ordinary social life. Sometimes these are called 'life-skills', and the possession of them helps to create a sense of 'self-esteem', which is currently a fashionable concept in the literature of health education. Clearly, like fitness, social well-being in this sense can be graded on a scale from negative to positive. It is a property of individuals and refers to their ability to cope in a social context—hence 'social well-being' is an appropriate term.

Can we link the absence of ill-health and the presence of well-being in a single concept of health in the manner of the WHO definition? This is not a rarefied question because it affects the legitimate scope of health education. If well-being is a component in the concept of health, then clearly health education has a much wider remit than it would otherwise have.

One important factor influencing this question is that ill-health and well-being cannot be related to each other as opposite poles on a linear scale. This approach has been tried by some theorists but it is not satisfactory, for it is logically possible (and not, in fact, uncommon) for someone to have poor physical health but a high state of well-being—as in the case of a terminal patient in a hospice, who is supported by caring staff and loving friends— or a good state of physical health but poor well-being—as in the case of someone who has no diseases or illnesses but lacks friends, a job, interests.

The fact that health (the absence of ill-health) and well-being cannot be related on a linear scale must raise the question of whether they are in fact two components of a single concept. It can be argued that they are aspects of a single concept.[16] But it may be preferable and less confusing conceptually to think of them as two overlapping concepts, rather than as a single concept with two dimensions. Thus the feeling of well-being that a person has after an invigorating swim can fairly be described as a 'glow of health', but the well-being or satisfaction that a person has after writing a chapter in a book, listening to a piece of music, or just playing an enjoyable game is less obviously related to concepts of health, and more obviously related to concepts such as 'enjoyment' and 'happiness'. Again, the well-being that is created by moving someone to better housing is more obviously related to concepts of 'welfare' than to that of health. The conclusion is that, while the concepts of health and well being overlap, they are distinct and cannot be combined into one concept. The point is succinctly put by Kenneth Boyd:

Disease is a medical category, while health is a moral category.[17]

But whether we think of health as a single multi-faceted concept, or as a narrower concept that overlaps with related concepts such as well-being and fitness, we must still examine two charges sometimes levelled at health promotional activities—that they are unethical in that they are 'imperialistic' and 'commercialize' health.

4.5.1 Imperialism

Those making the charge of health imperialism might argue that what in health promotion terms is 'positive health' is really just a name for a range of states, which are as easily or better seen in other ways. For example, 'well being' is just another name for happiness, and there are no professional skills that can reliably assist us to attain happiness. Again, the idea of 'fitness' might be said to be a technical one, relative to specific ends, such as playing in the Premier League, but not one with an important bearing on health. The charge of health imperialism can be directed also at mental health. Mental illness may satisfy some of the criteria for illness (although even that has been disputed), but positive mental health might be said by critics to be a concept that attempts to annex the territory of the well-adjusted to that of the healthy. For example, mental illnesses, such as depressions or obsessions, are incapacitating in a manner similar to that of physical illness, but to stress positive mental health might be seen as simply making a value judgement in favour of the conventional or the well-balanced as opposed to the eccentric.

In reply to this sort of objection, it is helpful to introduce the concept of health alliances. There are certain activities that are indisputably health promotion, but there are many others with which health promotion can form alliances. If health and health promotion can be seen in this logically and practically flexible way, then the charge of imperialism can be avoided.

4.5.2 Commercialism

The second ethical objection to health promotion is that it attempts to bypass autonomy and to sell health like a commodity. In this it might be said to resemble the advertisements for unhealthy products, which it is opposing.[18]

In reply to this argument we might question the premise that autonomy is something that everyone, in fact, possesses. People can be victims of all sorts of social processes and be lacking in power. For example, as the advertising of tobacco and alcohol becomes progressively more difficult in some countries, so the manufacturers have turned their attention to the developing world, and the huge markets that are opening up. As the countries become more affluent, so the consumption of such products increase with consequential long-term adverse health effects. Another example concerns breast-milk substitutes. All health authorities are clear about the value of breastfeeding for the mother and the baby. However, considerable pressure was brought to bear on mothers in developing countries to use breast-milk substitutes. Not only would this be more expensive, but the health benefits of breastfeeding would be lost. International action was required to deal with this issue. The WHO resolved that states ensure that there be no free or subsidized substitute, which would affect breastfeeding practice. This may seem to be merely a political compromise, but it may nevertheless be an effective way of implementing an ethically defensible position.

In view of the political and commercial power of the anti-health forces in society, health must be presented in as attractive a way as possible or health education will fail totally. If health educators confine themselves strictly to the rational, critical approach to education, then it is preferable to depict health education as an element within a larger health-promotion movement concerned with health advocacy, legislative change, fiscal reform, and the mobilization of community interests, as well as education narrowly conceived.

The tension between the ethical requirement to be person-respecting in methods, and the practical necessity to be effective, is addressed from an interesting point of view in the literature of self-help groups. The growth of self-care groups concerned with every conceivable malady, and involving both the sufferers and their relatives, has been a notable development during the last decade. These movements avoid the charge of paternalism commonly still made against every branch of health care, including health education. Apart from ethical considerations, self-care movements seem to be effective within their limits, although they may benefit from a professional health educator to advise and facilitate. Advising and facilitating is indeed an important role for health education.

4.6 'The organized efforts of society'

Public health medicine, according to the Acheson Report definition, must obtain its results 'through the organized efforts of society'. How are we to interpret this, and what ethical issues arise from our interpretation? Is it just a metaphor to speak of 'society' bringing about health? One obvious answer to this question is that to speak of 'society' bringing about health is a roundabout way of referring to our elected political representatives. We shall, therefore, begin by looking at the role of the state in health care, concentrating on health legislation.

4.6.1 Legislation and prevention

First, a person's right to exercise autonomy may be legitimately curtailed by health legislation when he or she is suffering from certain sorts of infectious disease or mental illness, such that the interests or health of others are liable to be harmed. There is no difficulty about the acceptance of this restriction in general terms. The problems arise over the more detailed application. For example, a topical question concerns the nature and extent of the restrictions that should be placed on sufferers from AIDS, or the extent of justifiable investigations or reporting of those who may be HIV-positive.[19] Again, it is controversial how far those who are mentally ill should be detained against their will, or what sort of treatment they should have if they are detained.

Pressure for legislation is generated as more becomes known about how diseases are transmitted. For example, the dangers of 'passive smoking' are now appreciated, and other sorts of environmental pollution are now known to cause or exacerbate diseases, such as asthma. There is, therefore, a case for curbing the freedom of both individuals and corporate bodies, such as industries, in the name of the autonomy of other individuals. This issue is, of course, a source of much political debate. Some countries have banned smoking in many public places, and various 'watch-dogs' keep a close eye on the consequences of the operation of the nuclear power industry. Although there can be political debate about applications of the 'preventing harm to others' idea, the general principle is clear and acceptable.

These problems become more acute when we consider the international dimension of health. In a developed country like the United Kingdom, international aspects have several implications. The first relates to communicable disease and, with the ease of transport now, the possibility of transmission to different populations becomes ever easier. Movement for business, leisure, or migration of populations is occurring on a scale as never before. The great plague, cholera, and influenza epidemics of the past, and AIDS, tuberculosis, and malaria in the present, show just how vulnerable the world is to such infections. The introduction of quarantine in Italy and France, in the fourteenth century, was one of the earliest attempts to control infections, and there is still ethical justification for certain sorts of boundary control for health reasons.

The need for international legislation is apparent also if we consider environmental issues, such as the radioactive release in Chernobyl. But environmental problems regularly cross international boundaries, as the effects of acid rain and global warming make clear. The need to ensure that there is an environmental impact assessment of economic growth has been set out in a series of programmes of 'sustainable development'.

4.6.2 Legislation and health promotion

Has the state any justification for using fiscal policy for passing legislation to promote positive health or well-being? A strong argument for maintaining that a government does have a duty to promote positive health can be found in the preamble to the Constitution of WHO,[20] which asserts that there is a right to positive health. In ambitious terms it states:

The enjoyment of the highest attainable standard of health is one of the fundamental rights of every human being without distinction of race, religion, political belief, economic or social condition.

If this is a fundamental right, then presumably there is a correlative duty laid upon governments to implement it. In other words, acceptance of the WHO Constitution commits states to health and welfare policies. How far such policies can be implemented no doubt turns on the wealth of the country, but there can be no doubt that wealthy Western nations are committed to implementing fiscal and legislative policies to enhance positive health.

To argue that there is a duty on governments to promote health for its own sake still leaves some questions unanswered. Supposing there is such a duty, can it be implemented other than at the expense of individual autonomy?

It is easy to slip into the error of regarding all legislation on the model of the criminal law—as restrictive prohibition backed by sanction. But this is an oversimplified way of looking at some health legislation. For example, legislation may require public bodies to make provision for the disabled. This is more aptly seen as positive creation of new opportunities than as negative prohibition. There are legal requirements on factory owners to restrict unpleasant pollutants, and on car manufacturers to ensure certain safety standards. Indeed, there is an enormous range of health legislation with a positive slant. Whereas this may diminish the freedom of some groups in society, it certainly extends the freedom of the majority and improves their quality of life.[21]

If we think of autonomy in this way, then health legislation is not *removing* our individual autonomy but rather *enhancing* it. In improving the general quality of life, legislation can add to our autonomy. This is obviously the case if we consider the example of provision for the disabled, but it is true also of anti-pollution legislation and many other types of health legislation.

4.6.3 Legislation and citizenship

So far in this section we have been concerned with the role of the state and health legislation. But there is much more to the 'organized efforts of society' than legislation. Let us state the five principles that the WHO[22] sees as the basis of health promotion:

1. Health promotion involves the population as a whole in the context of their everyday life, rather than focusing on people at risk for specific diseases.

2. Health promotion is directed towards action on the causes or determinants of health.

3. Health promotion combines diverse, but complementary methods or approaches, including communication, education, legislation, fiscal measures, organizational change, community development, and spontaneous local activities against health hazards.

4. Health promotion aims particularly at effective and concrete public participation.

5. While health promotion is basically an activity in the health and social fields, and not a medical service, health professionals—particularly in primary health care—have an important role in nurturing and enabling promotion.

How are we to interpret phrases such as 'concrete public participation'? What is the ethical importance of this approach?

One way of making sense of this idea is to think of society, not in terms of the individuals who make it up, but in terms of the institutions, practices, customs, political arrangements, and social class relationships that give structure to the society. From this point of view, people are related to each other by the structures of their society and, indeed, part of their identity is created by these social structures. We could then evaluate a society in terms of the way in which its social structures tend to produce health in the people who belong to that society. Just as we sometimes praise the 'atmosphere' in a school or hospital as one of well-being, so the social structures of an entire society might be said to make for or detract from health or well-being.

Some theorists with firm attachments to individualism might prefer to interpret what we have said as referring to health determinants, rather than health itself. For example, they might agree that a society with marked social class gradients, and corresponding gradients in the distribution of ill-health, is one with a tendency to create ill-health in individuals. Thus, in terms of this approach, if we speak of an 'unhealthy society' we are simply speaking metaphorically about the determinants, such as poor housing, and diet, and so on, that have helped to produce poor health states in individuals. Other thinkers might be prepared to extend language and to maintain that it is not a metaphor to characterize social relationships and structures as being themselves unhealthy. It is perhaps self-indulgent to pursue this theoretical question here, but it is certainly one way of making sense of the phrase 'the organized efforts of society', in the Acheson Report,[23] or 'effective and concrete public participation', as the WHO principle puts it.[24]

One context in which these phrases may have more practical meaning is that of rationing. Rationing will be discussed in detail in Chapter 5, but for present purposes we should note that there now seems to be a movement—famously initiated in the State of Oregon[25]—to involve the public in decisions about rationing health-care resources. One example of this is the use of 'citizens juries' in the Cambridge and Huntingdon Health Authority.[26] In a pilot scheme, a group of local people were recruited and met for 4 days to consider how priorities for rationing health care should be set and how far the public should be involved in these decisions. The discussions were mainly on matters of process but the project indicated a willingness amongst the public to be involved in matters of priority setting.

To the extent that there is exclusive emphasis on the state delivery of health care to individuals, there is the invitation to see health as a commodity to be supplied by the state. The same is true if we think of health as a commodity bought by private health insurance. But health is not in any sense a commodity. Health and well-being are in the end a set of relationships among citizens and the involvement of citizens in decisions about rationing is a good example. As Beauchamp[27] wrote:

Collective goods are ultimately a set of relationships among the citizens of a community, relationships in which the community as a whole participates to obtain desired benefits. These collective goods include aggregate states of welfare or well-being, including declining rates of disease and premature deaths; efforts to limit the resources society devotes to personal health services; shared and common access to a good, like medical care, to foster the sense of community and membership in the group itself. And finally, there are those highly important collective goods, shared or common beliefs and values.

It is clear that we can add a legal system to Beauchamp's list and, in particular, one designed to stimulate social responsibility. Indeed, it is plausible to suggest that the increasing government intervention on drunk-driving issues has encouraged a greater social awareness about the dangers of alcohol more generally, and thus a greater sense of community and individual responsibility. In a similar way, legislation designed to assist disabled or handicapped persons can also increase a sense of community responsibility for those groups. In other words, in so far as health legislation and other governmental health policies are directed at increasing community awareness, as distinct from being directed at the good of specific individuals, it is not paternalistic.

A health alliance, which has been shown to be helpful in developing community awareness, is that between health promotion services and community arts. Several projects have taken place and have had favourable evaluations. For example, the Bristol Area Specialist Health Promotion Service report on these projects—photography, the visual arts and drama.[28] Again, Bromley by Bow have on-going community arts and health projects.[29] The central message from these and similar projects is that disease and ill health cannot be eradicated by narrowly medical means; they must be tackled in a community context with the approval of the community. In other words, medicine needs health alliances, and the arts are a vital and ethically acceptable ally. The ancient Greeks recognized this when they made Apollo god of both medicine and the arts.

4.7 Evidence and judgement in public health

Public health medicine comprises a number of activities. Some of these depend on the evidence of epidemiology. But the gathering of this evidence, and deciding what to do with it, requires judgement, often social and political. The same is true of what is broadly called prevention. Health promotion, since it involves issues of well-being and lifestyle, relies heavily on moral judgement. Despite what some practitioners maintain it is essentially judgmental.

4.8 Conclusions

1. The evidence-base for public health medicine is epidemiology.

2. Judgement, especially ethical and political judgement, is essential not only for implementing policies based on epidemiology but also for deciding what studies are important to carry out.

3. Ethical judgement is equally integral in the prevention of disease, health promotion, and ensuring the organized efforts of society.

References

1. World Health Organization (WHO), *Constitution.* New York: WHO, 1946.
2. *Acheson Report. Public Health in England.* Report of the Committee of Inquiry into the future development of their public health function. London: HMSO, 1988.
3. Shy C, The failure of academic epidemiology: witness for the prosecution. *American Journal of Epidemiology* 1997; 145: 479–84.
4. Calman KC, Downie RS, Ethical principles and ethical issues in public health. In *Oxford Textbook of Public Health*, Vol. I (3rd edn). (ed. Detels R, Holland W, McEwen J, Omenn G). Oxford: Oxford University Press, 1997, pp.391–402.
5. Whitehead M, *The Concepts and Principles of Equity and Health.* WHO European Regional Office, 1990.
6. Omenn GS, Prevention and the elderly : what are the appropriate policies? *Health Affairs* 1990; 9: 80–93.
7. Charlton B, Public health medicine— a different kind of ethics? *Journal of the Royal Society of Medicine* 1993; 86: 194–5.
8. Kelly MP, Charlton B, Health promotion : time for a new philosophy? *BJGP* 1992; 42: 223–4.
9. Blaney R, Why Prevent Disease? In *Ethical Dilemmas in Health Promotion* (ed. Dioxiadis S). Chichester: John Wiley, 1987, pp.47–56.
10. Report of the working party on fluoridation of water and cancer : a review of the epidemiological evidence. London: HMSO, 1985.
11. Knox EG, Personal and public health care: conflict, congruence or accommodation? In *Ethical Dilemmas in Health Promotion* (ed. Dioxiadis S). Chichester: John Wiley, 1987, pp.59–68.
12. Knox, op. cit., pp.59–68.
13. Stone S, Stewart S, *Towards a Screening Strategy for Scotland.* Scottish Forum for Public Health Medicine, Glasgow, 1994.
14. Shickle D, Shandwick R, The ethics of screening : is 'screeningitis' an incurable disease? *Journal of Medical Ethics* 1994; 20: 12–8.

15. World Health Organisation (WHO) *Constitution* New York: WHO, 1946.
16. Downie RS, Tannahill C, Tannahill A, *Health Promotion : Models and Values* (2nd edn). Oxford: Oxford University Press, 1996.
17. Boyd KM, Health care ethics, health and disease. In *Principles of Health Care Ethics* (ed. Gillon R). Chichester: Wiley, 1994, pp.807–17
18. Williams G. Health Promotion - caring concern or slick salesmanship? *Journal of Medical Ethics* 1984; 10: 191–5.
19. Walters L, Ethical issues in the prevention and treatment of HIV infection and AIDS. *Science* 1988; 239: 597–603.
20. WHO, 1946, op. cit., preamble.
21. Pinet G, Health legislation, prevention and ethics. In *Ethical Dilemmas in Health Promotion* (ed. Dioxiadis S). Chichester: John Wiley, 1987, pp.83–97.
22. WHO. Health promotion : a discussion document on the concepts and principles. Copenhagen: WHO, 1984.
23. Acheson Report, op. cit., p.1.
24. WHO, 1984 op. cit., pp.27–31.
25. Smith R, Rationing health care: moving the debate forward. *BMJ* 1996; 312: 1311–2.
26. Lenaghan J, New B, Mitchell E, Setting priorities: is there a role for citizens' juries? *BMJ* 1996; 312: 1553–4.
27. Beauchamp D, Lifestyle, public health and paternalism. In *Ethical Dilemmas in Health Promotion* (ed. Dioxiadis S). Chichester: John Wiley, 1987, p.72.
28. Hecht R (ed.) *I Talk Now*. Bristol Specialist Health Promotion Service, Central Health Clinic, Bristol, 1996.
29. Bromley by Bow Centre Annual Report 1995–96. London: Bromley By Bow, 1996.

Editors' note to Chapter 5

To illustrate the applicability of our central thesis—that evidence and judgement form a seamless garment—we invited a hospital consultant to consider how far this thesis might be relevant to a currently controversial area of health care: resource management, prioritizing, or rationing. We are particularly grateful to Dr Fiona Randall for agreeing to write this chapter. First, she is able to offer the perspective of a hospital consultant, and it is hospital consultants who are perhaps most aware of resource constraints. Second, we were interested to see how our general line of argument would work out in an area at the rock-face of current controversy. Her views on this important topic are much wider than can be expressed within the constraints we have imposed on her. No doubt she will have occasion to publish a more extended version of them.

RSD
RJM

5 Judgement and resource management

FIONA RANDALL

5.1 The necessity for rationing

Resource management, or prioritizing, or rationing in health care is an imposed distribution system that has two goals: first, to ensure the best use of resources by using the most cost-effective treatments; and second, to ensure a just or fair distribution of treatment benefits. Rationing takes place at two levels: macro-allocation, where budgets are allocated for the treatments of different diseases, and for medical and nursing care; and micro-allocation, where discrimination between individual patients is necessary because it is not possible to give the most beneficial care or treatment to every patient. Obviously major moral and practical problems arise at both levels. Nevertheless, it will be the contention of this chapter that a rationing system is required now and will continue to be required in the future. To maintain such a position with any hope of plausibility, we must examine both the evidence on which a system of rationing might be based, and the sorts of judgement necessary to implement it.

The ways in which rationing can be implemented will obviously vary to some extent, depending on the particular system of health-care delivery and financing that is operative. But many of the broad principles are the same, so while my discussion is centred on the UK National Health Service (NHS), I hope that my arguments will be more widely applicable. It should also be noted that some writers in this area, and all politicians, prefer the terms 'resource management' or 'prioritizing' to the term 'rationing'. I do not distinguish between them, and will now move to outlining the bearing of evidence on rationing.

Evidence from clinical trials will yield information about the outcomes of treatment in terms of health benefits, harms, and risks. Economic assessment will tell us how much treatments cost in terms of human and financial resources. Evidence regarding the net benefits of treatments and care is essential for rationing decisions. It is naive to think that the most effective treatments will cost less to provide, or that health-care costs will decrease as life-prolonging treatments enable people to live longer. The image of health care enabling the majority of people to live healthy and independent lives until their tenth decade, when they die after a very short illness, is exceedingly likely to be a mirage. Constraints of financial and human resources will always exist, especially in a health service that is necessarily cash-limited because it is funded by taxation. Patients' capacity to benefit from treatment and care will always exceed the possible supply of treatment and care. In the clinical context, the public, patients, and health-care professionals will expect and demand treatment and care, and it will not be possible to meet all of their expectations and demands. Whilst evidence will give us more information about the effects of treatment, it cannot tell us how the benefits of treatment should be distributed; judgement is required for that.

5.2 Financial and justice arguments for rationing

I am discussing the financial and the justice arguments for rationing in the same section because they run together and it is artificial to separate them. I shall try to make clear how they are linked.

The facts of the case are clear—both medical technology and care require financial and human resources, which in the United Kingdom are limited. Financial resources are provided through taxation and charitable contribution, and human resources by the education and funding of health-care professionals. Medical technology is becoming ever more expensive, ever more capable of prolonging life for a little longer, often able to make life more comfortable in the face of illness, and very occasionally able to find new cures for hitherto incurable and fatal illness. As affluent Western populations live longer to develop degenerative diseases, they are likely to need more care just to fulfil the activities of daily living—keeping warm, being fed, moving around the house. Even if taxation were increased to provide a greater fund for medical technology and care, and even if it were possible to fund and maintain a larger workforce of health carers, demand would always exceed supply. It is not possible now, and never will be possible, to provide all the treatment and care that would be of benefit to the population. Therefore, some people inevitably will be denied care and treatment from which they could benefit. It is this fact that the public, patients, and health-care professionals find most difficult to accept and which causes them to try to deny the fact that rationing is morally necessary and to evade attempts at implementing it.

Two possible mechanisms for attempting to avoid rationing are sometimes suggested: first, increasing public funding, for example, through increasing income tax; and second, through narrowing the boundaries of 'health care'. Although the first suggestion would enable more treatments and care to be provided within the budget for health care, demand will exceed supply for the foreseeable future. The capacity of patients to benefit from medical technology is increasing constantly as research reveals more ways to provide health benefits, and similarly the capacity of patients to benefit from care is increasing constantly as we enable people to live longer.

The second suggestion seems more promising. Setting limits to, or redefining what, the NHS should provide are necessary procedures whatever health service a country provides for its population. A process of continually narrowing the scope of health care to be provided would reduce health-care costs. For example, in the UK the elderly who require 24-hour nursing care no longer have this care provided free of charge in a long-stay hospital. Instead, they have to fund their own care in privately owned nursing homes if they have more than a modest amount of savings. Yet even this very significant narrowing of NHS provision, which has reduced costs to the health service, has not enabled sufficient funds to be available to provide all the treatment and care from which patients could benefit. Even if there were a continuous process of setting ever greater limits to the scope of NHS provision, financial constraints would still exist. Moreover, as I shall later argue, reducing the scope of the health service is itself a disguised form of rationing.

Health-care professionals, the public, and politicians, need to be reminded of the consequences of *not* rationing health care. I have said that rationing is an externally imposed distribution system which endeavours to derive the greatest benefit from medical technology and care and to distribute that benefit in a way that is as just and fair as possible. If health-care rationing is not undertaken, then it is very clear that we will not make the best use of resources, and unjust distribution of health-care benefits will occur. For example, a fixed annual budget commencing in April may well be spent by December, so should people becoming ill in January be denied treatment or care? This consequence would be very unjust. Are those patients, whose doctors spend money regardless of budgetary constraints, to have the expensive treatments, while patients of other doctors, who respect budget constraints, to lose out because money has to be taken from their budgets to meet the shortfall created by the overspending doctors? This too sounds most unjust, particularly as patients may be denied treatments that are more beneficial in order to fund treatments that are less beneficial. Failure to ration health care will lead to less than optimal use of resources in that it may lead to the carrying out of treatments with only marginal benefits, and in being random in its distribution of treatments and care, it will also be unjust.

Rationing is necessary so that each person has the best chance of obtaining optimal treatment when he or she becomes ill. People behind a 'veil of ignorance' would wish to dwell in a community where the best use was made of health care funded by that community, and where benefits were fairly distributed. Politicians, health-care professionals, and the public, will need to be continuously reminded of this fact in order to bolster their determination and courage to formulate and implement rationing policies. The community as a whole needs, first, to believe in the practical reality of capacity-for-benefit exceeding supply, and, second, to believe in the importance of justice in the use of public resources for health care.

Our conclusion then is that it is necessary to have a system of rationing, and one which produces just outcomes, or at least outcomes less unjust than those described above. It is financially necessary, in that governments of countries in industrialized nations have now realized that their populations will not support significantly increased taxation to provide ever-increasing funding for health services. It is morally necessary, in that we should neither tolerate nor turn a blind eye to the unjust outcomes described.

This conclusion, of course, does not answer the question of who should ration. We can predict that politicians will continue to pass the responsibility for rationing to health-care professionals. Yet this may be preferable to a situation where those unfamiliar with the benefits and harms of treatments have the authority and power to allocate resources. On the other hand, the relative value of various health benefits, and relative disvalue of various harms of treatments, are judgements that, it may be argued, should be taken on a public scale, and should be subject to public consultation. After all, health care exists for the public, and the public fund it, so their views of the relative values of benefits and disvalue of harms should be sought. Health-care professionals may, because of their work, have a slanted and unrepresentative view. Health-care professionals and the public should both be involved in formulating rationing policies. Such policies would then need to be ratified by government—this step could prove problematic as politicians would not wish to be seen as restricting care or treatment options.

5.3 Doctors' objections to rationing

Before we can expect doctors to believe in the necessity for rationing we must meet two arguments commonly used by doctors against the need for rationing, or at least against their involvement in the process. These are the 'clinical freedom' argument and the 'patient's best interests' argument.

Clinical freedom is the notion that a doctor should be free to provide whatever treatment he or she considers to be in the best interest of a particular patient. It is a strongly held ideal, and some doctors might even regard it as some sort of right. Thus they might regard the right to prescribe as they consider best for the patient to override other considerations, such as the welfare of other patients or the community.

Clinical freedom obviously can never be absolute; it must always be constrained by law. Let us assume that clinical freedom is similar to the idea of freedom in a democratic society. In a democratic society it is considered right that people should be free to pursue their own ideals and life plans provided they function within the law. Yet even in a democracy there are limits to personal freedom. These limits may be imposed by law. For example, we have to pay taxes, obey speed limits, and wear seatbelts in cars. These limits are necessary if we are to live together successfully and safely in a community. There are also moral limits to personal freedom. We should not do things that harm others, even if such actions are not proscribed by law. Such limits are 'imposed' by the moral law. In a similar way, the freedom of clinicians ought to be limited by the law and by the majority opinion of their informed colleagues in other specialties and by team members. I shall later (Section 5.4) develop the communitarian idea of the team as a constraint on individual clinical freedom. In the meantime, I am by no means suggesting the removal of clinical freedom but only its responsible use in a team spirit.

It should also be noted that, 'Granting physicians clinical autonomy is justified by reference to the patient's interests, not the physician's'.[1] Thus the foundation of the concept of clinical freedom or autonomy for physicians is the good of patients, not physicians. So the interpretation of the meaning of clinical freedom must be made in the context of the good of patients, which means patients in a general sense rather than just one particular patient in front of just one particular physician. In other words, the 'clinical freedom' argument against rationing is really secondary to the 'patient's best interests' argument, and I shall, therefore, turn to consider it.

Doctors who believe that they have a single or overriding obligation to do the best for the patient before them, regardless of the resource consequences, tend to argue that the nature of the special relationship between them and that patient requires that they do not in any way compromise that patient's interests, even in the interests of other patients.

How plausible is the 'special relationship' argument? It can be interpreted in two ways. In terms of the first way, which we can call the 'advocacy' interpretation of the special relationship, the doctor should be loyal to his individual patients and advocate their best interests. But in terms of this interpretation, duties of advocacy or of loyalty cannot override duties of general justice. Take an analogous case. A wife has duties of loyalty and advocacy with respect to the interests of her husband, but if she happens to discover that her husband is a child-molester, then the duty of general justice, to have his activities stopped even at the cost of going to the police, overrides the duties of advocacy and loyalty.

There is, however, a second interpretation of the special relationship between doctor and patient. It might be argued that the special relationship is more like a promissory relationship. If A promises B some goods or service, it is not at all obvious that a duty of general justice will override this. In a similar way, it might be claimed that the doctor's special relationship to his patient is one of special justice, like a kind of promise to do his best for that patient, and not the generality of patients. How are we to interpret the special relationship: as one of 'advocacy' or as one of 'special justice'?

It might be said that the question is artificial because there are elements of both advocacy and special justice in the doctor–patient relationship. But rather than enter into this debate, we can move the argument on by asking the question: who is the doctor's patient? To put it another way, to whom does a doctor have positive duties to act 'in the patient's best interests'? Do doctors have a special relationship and obligations to benefit just the patient in front of them at an instant, or equally to all their patients? Do they owe obligations to all the people from the community who are patients of that NHS Trust (in the case of hospital doctors) or primary care group (in the case of general practitioners).

No one contests the fact that the doctor–patient relationship confers on the doctor a responsibility to do the best possible in the circumstances for the patient in front of him. But what of all the other patients he will have the same obligation towards during the rest of the financial year? They are also his patients, present before him on different occasions, so surely he must have an equal obligation to do the best possible for each patient at whatever time in the year the referral takes place. So, if the doctor's budget is a fixed constraint and is to be respected as such, and assuming insufficient resources are available to provide all the care and treatment that would be beneficial, then care and treatment must be rationed at the level of the individual patient in order to ensure that patients coming forward at the end of the year can be treated as well as patients at the beginning of the year.

In other words, since all patients referred to a single consultant or attending a general practitioner during a year are owed a fair share of that doctor's resources, rationing is essential at the level of the individual patient. Thus, rationing is required between patients, even though there is no doubt that the doctor has a special responsibility towards all of them arising from the professional relationship with each. This is the same as pointing out that there is a necessity to ration treatment and care provision amongst current patients, a policy that is generally accepted. For example, if on a particular day two patients would benefit from a particular resource (such as a bed on the coronary care unit) but it is available only for one, then rationing at the individual patient level is required, and this form of rationing is widely accepted as justifiable. One patient will receive a higher standard of treatment than the other, and usually doctors react to this decision dilemma by giving the specialist bed to the patient who is likely to derive most benefit from it.

We can provide a summing up of this argument in terms of the use of the apostrophe 's': we hold that doctors must base their treatments decisions not on the '*patient's* best interests' but on the '*patients*' best interests'! This moves our argument towards a consideration of the responsibility of a hospital staff or primary care group as a team towards the community they serve.

5.4 Team responsibility and health professionals as trustees

The present politically driven initiative within the UK National Health Service is gradually attempting to devolve responsibility for deciding what health care should be provided to groups of general practices called primary care groups (or local health-care co-operatives in Scotland). The problem with rationing at the level of the primary care group is that it seems very difficult for members of different practices to agree on treatment priorities and rationing policies. Moreover, it is very difficult for members of one practice to alter the behaviour of members of another practice who are not adhering to the rationing policy agreed by the majority and are, therefore, overspending. No-one seems to know what will happen if a primary care group becomes significantly overspent. Unfortunately it seems likely that in order to remain in budget for the financial year, treatment that is clearly beneficial and normally routinely available would have to be denied to some patients. Whilst the authority and responsibility for rationing seems gradually to be passing to primary care groups, they do not appear to have a mechanism for enforcing inevitable and necessary rationing policies on their members. This situation is likely to lead to low morale and bad feeling between practitioners, and could result in the group giving up attempts to constrain costs with disastrously unjust consequences for some patients.

If treatment priorities are decided by primary care groups, it is very likely that different groups will assign different priorities to different treatments. It then follows that whether a treatment is available will depend on the opinion of the patient's primary care group and thus, ultimately, on where the patient lives. The same result occurs where health authorities have to decide on treatment priorities. This has been referred to as 'rationing by post code' and is widely accepted to be an unjust outcome in a publicly funded health service. The only solution would be to decide at national level the 'illnesses' that the NHS will treat, and also to decide at national level which drugs will be available and purchased by the NHS for certain conditions. The National Institute for Clinical Excellence (NICE) has been set up to fulfil this role. However, rationing criteria will have no success unless there are very strong incentives, be they legal or moral, or preferably both, for doctors and other health-care professionals to implement the rationing system once it has been agreed, and even if they personally feel that some patients will be disadvantaged in order that others can benefit.

The functional economic unit of secondary health care is now the NHS Hospital Trust. The budget for the secondary care of a community is given to that Trust, and extra money is provided if care has to be provided for a patient not resident in the specified catchment area of the Trust. Each consultant is a member of a team of consultants (and other health professionals) caring for a community as a joint responsibility. The team of health-care professionals within the Trust, with the organizational assistance of management staff, have the task of providing the best possible care for the people living in the catchment area within the budget. The budget is currently provided largely by the health authority, but in the future it may increasingly be controlled by primary care groups.

Consultants in the NHS are all team members, not isolated doctors whose only responsibility is towards the patient in front of them. This is because no single consultant could provide the patient's care without the involvement of a host of colleagues in a variety of departments in the Trust. Since consultants can fulfil their function only in the context of team functioning, it follows that there is a responsibility to work as a member of that team. This entails not exploiting other departments by regarding them as a means to obtain extra funding to bail out an overspend in one's own department.

Thus consultants should be good team players in terms of co-operating with their professional colleagues to make the most just use, and the best use, of the resources available for the community served by the NHS Trust. There is a moral obligation to strive for this goal. Rationing is essential to achieve it. So rationing activities are not simply financially justifiable: they are morally required of NHS consultants.

Refusal to take joint responsibility for the implementation of agreed rationing policies within the Trust is very likely to result in an unjust distribution of resources, which consequence is morally unacceptable. Therefore, any refusal to participate in implementing agreed rationing policies must be based on a reasonable claim that one's own action will result in a use of resources, which is not simply better in health benefit terms, but is also as just or more just than that attainable via the existing rationing policy. Maverick overspending without regard for the consequences to other patients in that community cannot be justified morally.

One might argue that as a team member a consultant should implement a rationing policy, which has been agreed within the Trust team, even though he or she believes the policy to be less just than could be achieved. Teamwork requires respect for team decisions, even though the individual may at times disagree with them.

Implementing a rationing policy may mean rationing at the level of individual patients (micro-allocation), so that some patients are given the expensive treatment that is denied to other patients, or it may mean agreeing not to provide an expensive treatment that the Trust team or the Health Authority has decided cannot be made available to any patients following a cost/benefit analysis (macro-allocation).

In the context of either a primary care group or an NHS hospital Trust, health-care professionals should regard NHS resources as having been given to them in trust for the health care of the community. The health-care professionals are like trustees of a charity, whose responsibility is to make the best use of the charity's resources and distribute the benefits justly. In effect, all health-care professionals, administrative, and management staff, within a primary care group or hospital Trust, are trustees.

A more detailed account of how health care might be rationed requires a development of the distinction we have already touched on, between macro-allocation and micro-allocation. Macro-allocation requires us to decide which services and treatments a publicly funded health service should provide. Micro-allocation requires us to decide which patients should receive these treatments or services. Let us consider these separately.

5.5 Macro-allocation: some concepts

A publicly funded health service exists to provide health benefits. However, virtually all treatment and care options entail some harms (side-effects and inconveniences) and some risks. Decisions regarding which treatments and care facilities a publicly funded health service should provide require consideration of the benefits, harms, and risks of each treatment or care option, and also the costs of those options. Some concepts have been central to discussions regarding which treatments and care should be provided. Let us examine some of these.

There have been many attempts to define 'health'.[2] However, a universally acceptable definition of health—even if it could be established—would not decide those benefits that a publicly funded service should provide. Such a decision is essentially a moral judgement and the act of choosing a definition of health does not in itself make clear which services should be provided.

Similar considerations apply to the concept of need, used as a basis for macro-allocation. The concept of need in health care is generally taken to imply a strong moral 'ought' or duty on behalf of an affluent society to meet that need. Thus it may be thought that if we could adequately describe what we mean by 'need', we would achieve a description of those benefits that the health service ought to provide. However, as with the concept of health, the way we decide to describe the concept of need will not in itself make clear what services should be provided by publicly funded health care. For example, if we take a narrow view of the concept of need, we might say that a need is 'something without which one will be fundamentally harmed', as has been suggested by Beauchamp and Childress.[3] In the context of health care, this definition would imply that we might need health care that would prolong life, or alleviate incapacitating suffering or disability. But it is less clear that a desire to have a child constitutes a need which if not satisfied will fundamentally harm us. It is even more debatable whether counselling after the breakdown or loss of a relationship constitutes a need in this sense.

Some have suggested a much broader definition, and have defined need as 'capacity to benefit'.[4] According to this definition, people need from the health services everything that could benefit their health. This would entail very regular investigation and treatment of any factor, such as blood pressure and serum lipids, control of which would have a beneficial effect on health. It would also entail the idea that everyone needs to be assured of good housing, lack of deprivation, rewarding employment, and a healthy lifestyle, and that such benefits should be provided as part of a health-care package. If we were to provide everything that would benefit the health of each individual, the responsibilities of the health service would need to be infinite. Moreover, it is interesting to note that, with regard to other public services, such as education and housing, we do not consider that the publicly funded service should provide everything from which each individual could benefit.

If the use of such essentially contestable concepts, such as health, need, and so on, cannot provide solutions to the problems of macro-allocation, then we must turn to direct consideration of the many benefits derived from available treatments and care packages. We must try to evaluate the net benefits from treatment and care options by weighing up the magnitude and likelihood of the benefits against the magnitude and likelihood of harms and risks of those options. Having established the nature and magnitude of the net benefits, we are left with the task of deciding which of those benefits ought to be provided by the publicly funded service.

5.6 Macro-allocation: the QALY

Health care occurs via a *process*, which may in itself be beneficial or harmful. For example, the process of chemotherapy for curative treatment of malignancies is very unpleasant owing to the side-effects of drugs, possible need for isolation, altered body image due to hair loss, etc. People are willing to undergo this very unpleasant and harmful process only because of the possibility of cure. In this case, the process of treatment is not beneficial. On the other hand, the process of treatment and care may be beneficial. For example, in the context of palliative care, excellent physical care and symptom control performed compassionately may allay patients' fears, and the reduction in anxiety may significantly reduce symptoms, such as pain and dyspnoea. Similarly, it could be argued that the benefit of care for the physically or mentally frail elderly actually arises from the process of care itself.

Although it is acknowledged that the process of treatment and care may itself be harmful or beneficial, when macro-allocation of resources is undertaken it is usually only the *outcome* of care or treatment that is considered. Clearly this is a morally unsatisfactory situation. At this stage in the discussion we should simply note the importance of assessing the benefits, harms, and risks of the process of health care.

The most sustained and serious attempt to asses the benefits and harms arising from health care has been the development of the concept of the 'Quality Adjusted Life Year' or QALY. This is an attempt to express all the outcomes of health care in common units called QALYs. The view is that health has two main dimensions: length and quality. Effective health care must either extend life or improve its quality, or preferably both, so in theory all effective health care will produce Quality Adjusted Life Years or QALYs.[5]

Of course evidence can and will demonstrate the time-span by which a treatment prolongs life, be it days, months, or years. There is no moral or practical problem with the concept of added time to life, measured in our standard units of time. However, there are both moral and practical problems with the idea of assessing the *quality of life* change, which results from treatment, and then with expressing that quality as a numerical value on a metrical scale. Yet this is exactly what is central to the concept of the QALY. The quality of life of the health state before and after treatment is represented as a number on a scale. The scale used to represent the quality of the patient's life before and after treatment ranges from 0.0 to 1.0, where 1.0 represents full health and 0.0 represents no quality of life, or death. According to the QALY concept, it is possible to be in a health state whose quality of life is rated as worse than death (some may consider persistent vegetative state, advanced dementia, or quadriplegia to be worse than death). A quality of life worse than death would be measured as a minus figure, e.g. -0.5. The figures on the scale for each health state are derived by questioning either the general public, those living in the health states, or health professionals. It is apparent that it may be of crucial importance which group is assessing the quality of life in each health state.

To calculate the health gain or QALYs from a particular treatment, the number of years by which life is prolonged is multiplied by the improvement in quality of life resulting from the treatment. For example, if a coronary bypass graft added 10 years to the patient's life, at a health state rated as 0.9, then the outcome of the treatment is 9 QALYs. Similarly, if a treatment prolonged life for 5 years but in a state of paraplegia rated as 0.5 on the quality of life scale, then the QALYs gained would be only 2.5. It can be seen that the underlying assumption of the QALY is that people are likely to prefer a shorter life of high quality, rather than a longer life of low quality.

Whilst it is conceptually easy to calculate QALYs for treatments that do actually prolong life, it is much less apparent how this can be done for treatments (such as artificial hip replacement) that do not prolong life at all but which improve its quality. The QALY score for such treatments is achieved by making an assumption about the patient's expected length of life, say 10 years, and multiplying this by the improvement in quality. For example, if quality is improved from 0.7 to 0.9, and the patient lives for 10 years, the QALY gain as an outcome of hip replacement is 0.2×10 or 2 QALYs.

Logically it would seem that the calculations must become more complex where a treatment both prolongs life and improves its quality at the same time. For example, a coronary artery bypass graft performed on an elderly person may prolong life for only 4 years, but may improve quality of life from the initial health state. We need not concern ourselves with the complexities of such calculations. Rather, we should question whether they actually give us a more accurate impression of health gain, than if the person's state before and after the bypass graft were just *described* to us, together with relevant *evidence* about the expected prolongation of life in years

Many criticisms have been made of the concept of the QALY and of its use in macro-allocation. However, the single and most important criticism is that it simply is not possible to place a numerical value on quality of life of health states, where the number is part of a metrical scale. There are two reasons for this.

First, there is no clear and universally accepted concept of quality of life. For example, 'quality' may be thought to lie in happiness, in being able to work, in the ability to choose, or in membership of a community, to name but a few candidates![6] When people are asked to rate the quality of life of a particular health state on a numerical scale, we have no idea what concept of quality of life is in their minds. If they rate the quality of life in a wheelchair as 0.5, we do not know if this is because they believe a paraplegic person cannot hold down a satisfying job, or have satisfactory relationships in the community, or have an adequate range of life choices, or is simply very unhappy for any reason.

Second, when they are asked to rate quality of life on a scale from 0.0 to 1.0, they are really placing health states in a series, or producing a 'rational ordering' of those health states. They are not necessarily saying that a quality of life of 0.6 is twice as good as one of 0.3 (see Section 1.7.3). They are considering the rank ordering of health states. It is exceedingly unlikely that they are wondering whether all the intervals on the scale are separated by the same amount. It is possible that they are actually rating quality of life on a scale more like a logarithmic scale, such as the Richter scale used to measure earthquakes. There are simply no grounds for assuming that they are either able to rate quality of life on a metrical scale or that they are actually doing so. Since this assumption is not well founded, the entire logical and arithmetical foundation of the QALY concept fails.

If the use of the scale to describe quality of life is invalid, then the use of that measure in a calculation to describe the benefit of health interventions as a single figure simply confounds the errors. When data are being handled to achieve a goal, it is often said 'rubbish in, rubbish out'. In other words, if the data put into the equation are invalid, so will be the result. The problem in the QALY system is that if rubbish is put in, something even worse than rubbish will be put out, for there is a real risk that the error in estimate of quality of life will literally be multiplied. This would lead to counter-intuitive, if not disastrously misleading, results in terms of QALYs gained by the majority of treatments.

Most of the other criticisms of QALYs are based on the judgement that they appear to produce conclusions regarding macro-allocation, which are *intuitively* either unwise or unjust. For example, it has been suggested that these problems can all be solved by 'weighting' the QALY score in a certain direction, so as to make the result more intuitively acceptable. For example, a higher number of QALYs would always be obtained for curative treatment of life-threatening conditions in young people than for curative treatment of similar conditions for older people, since more years of life would be gained. If allocation of health-care resources followed this conclusion the result would be pervasive discrimination against older people as a group. It has been suggested that the QALY result should be manipulated mathematically (referred to as 'weighting') in order to prevent this result.

A second counter-intuitive result of QALY calculations would be the very low priority given to palliative care when the patient is known to be terminally ill. Any treatment that does not prolong life for the dying patient, but which improves its quality for the short time remaining, will produce a very low QALY score and will therefore not be funded. Yet good relief of distress at the end of life, or 'dying well', is generally thought to be a high priority. The counter-intuitive conclusion of the QALY calculation could be altered mathematically by positively weighting the quality of life in the last few weeks or months. However, the weighting required to make any palliative care available at all following QALY calculations would have to be very significant!

Obviously it is possible mathematically to manipulate QALY scores in order to obtain results that are not counter-intuitive in terms of macro-allocation. However, we must ask what is the point? If QALY scores produce conclusions for macro-allocation that are deemed intuitively to be unjust, then it would be more rational to abandon the QALY concept because experiments using it have produced unacceptable results rather than to continue to massage the figures to obtain the results which we thought were just in the first place.

The application of humane clinical judgement to these kinds of situations has shown that the QALY concept has fundamental flaws. We cannot rate the quality of life of a health state on a numerical scale (Section 1.7.3). Therefore, any form of numerical trade-off between length of life and quality of life is not possible. If tried, it yields results that are not only meaningless but also lead to conclusions about macro-allocation which are counter-intuitive. The benefits of prolonging life and decreasing distress due to disease are incommensurable and cannot be evaluated numerically, either individually or on some sort of global quality of life scale. Thus they should simply be described qualitatively.

In other words, economic or mathematical data require to be corrected by clinical judgement. The need for clinical judgement cannot be eliminated in medicine by pseudo-technicalities.

5.7 How should macro-allocation decisions be made?

Macro-allocation decisions are to do with what treatments and care the publicly funded health care service should provide, and how much of them. We have said that these decisions entail discrimination between treatments or services. We can also say that the benefits of health care fall into three categories: first, the prolongation of life; second, the relief of distressing symptoms arising from physical and mental illness; and third, care and assistance with the activities of daily living when this becomes necessary because of physical disability or mental infirmity.

When macro-allocation decisions are made the following are the most relevant considerations that will affect judgement:

(1) the characteristics of the population and the community to be served;

(2) the characteristics of the various treatments and services;

(3) moral principles of justice.

1. Macro-allocation decisions must depend on the relevant characteristics of the population and the context of the community. For example, in the midst of a war associated with casualties and food shortages, no-one would wish to argue that setting up screening programmes to prevent malignant disease late in life should be a high priority in health care. Economically deprived nations will naturally prioritize provision of adequate food, warmth, shelter, and hygiene to enable the population to survive, and simple and cheap preventive measures against infectious diseases. They are unable to afford more expensive life-prolonging treatments, such as renal dialysis, anti-viral treatment for AIDS or palliative treatments for malignant disease. It would clearly be wrong to spend money on such treatments rather than providing the basics of food and inexpensive vaccinations and antibiotics.

2. Where services are to be considered, such as a screening service, immunization services, or the provision of free nursing care to those dependant on such care, then the costs and the benefits of the service to the community and to the individuals who receive it are all relevant.

There may be considerable difficulty in deriving information regarding benefit from the existing evidence base. For example, nursing care is not free to all and has not been so for some time, so we have no evidence about its benefit to individuals, although we might argue for its likely benefits. The long-term outcomes of screening programmes are also unknown at this time, and the best we can do is to extrapolate from the information we have. In assessing costs and benefits, the number of people to whom the service is given is relevant—if a large number will receive it then the costs may be high but the total benefit is also likely to be large.

Where treatments are concerned, roughly the same considerations apply. The benefits, harms and risks of the process of care during the treatment, which will include the possible side-effects and mishaps, should be described. The outcomes of the treatment should also be examined. The evidence from research will obviously be crucial in providing the information base for these assessments. As we have seen, attempts to quantify net benefit and to represent it as a single numerical figure in a scale are invalid. In particular, we should reject numerical scores for quality of life during and after treatment as an assessment of benefit, since these are invalid, i.e. cannot measure what they are said to measure (Section 5.6). Therefore, qualitative descriptions of benefit are to be preferred. The exception to this general rule would occur where there is evidence regarding the length by which life has been prolonged by a treatment, since this can be represented in units of time and is valid as such. Harms and risks should be described qualitatively also for the same reasons.

3. Equity is the principle of fairness or justice in the distribution of benefits and burdens in a community. It naturally, and rightly, comes to mind when considering the distribution of the benefits of publicly funded health care. Aristotle originally described equity in his formal principle of justice, which states that equals

should be treated equally, and unequals, unequally in proportion to their relevant inequality.[7] This means that we should treat people in the same way (equally) unless there are relevant differences between them.

Efficiency (or sometimes the concept of utility is used here) is to do with attaining the maximum output from the input of resources. However, it is necessary to specify the precise goal of efficiency—in other words, exactly what output is to be maximized from the resources. For example, if the goal of efficiency (the output to be maximized) is QALYs, then efficiency would mean simply producing the maximum QALYs from a unit of input of resources. If one such unit could yield 10 QALYs for one person or 1 QALY each for seven people, then if QALYs are the goal of efficiency, one must give the unit of resources to the one person who gains 10 QALYs, whilst the seven people die. On the other hand, if the goal of efficiency is the maximum number of people whose life could be extended, one should use the one unit of resource to prolong the life of seven people for 1 year each. It can be seen that in judging the efficiency of various macro-allocation strategies, one must be specific about what the goal of efficiency or the output to be maximized is.

Other moral principles frequently used in discussing health-care, such as the importance of obtaining consent and respecting the patient's refusal of treatment, or beneficence and non-maleficence, are more relevant to the problems of micro-allocation, and we shall note their force in that context.

In concluding this very brief account of macro-allocation, I am suggesting that equal access to a decent minimum of health care should be available for everyone. In order to fund this, efficient use of health care resources is required. Judgements about efficiency cannot be made unless one specifies the precise goal of the efficiency drive. Maximizing the chosen health benefit per unit of resource will necessitate restriction of choices for patients and professionals.

The macro-allocation judgements that a community makes and the policies it follows reflect the relative values attributed by that community to the three major types of benefits gained from health care. Those relative values also tell us something about the attitudes of members of that society to those vulnerable people who are dependent on others for care. Perhaps they also tell us something about attitudes towards death and the degree of acceptance of our inescapable human mortality. It is possible that by influencing and altering macro-allocation policies those responsible for making them may be able to influence society's attitudes to vulnerable people, and perhaps also towards death itself. Thus it can be argued that macro-allocation strategies can be a force for either good or evil.

5.8 Micro-allocation

The necessity to discriminate between individuals in order to determine who receives the greater share of scarce resources is an unpleasant and unavoidable reality. Unfortunately, however hard we try to establish macro-allocation policies that will diminish the necessity to discriminate between individuals, such discrimination will remain an inescapable and very difficult task for health-care professionals. This is a sphere in which judgement is necessary. In particular, just as in macro-allocation there must be a balance between the moral principles of equity and efficiency or utility, so in micro-allocation there must be a balance between the principles of non-maleficence, beneficence, respect for the patient's consent to, or refusal of, treatment, equity, and efficiency.

For example, it will always be necessary for professionals to decide how to divide the precious resource of their time between patients (or increasingly, between patients and relatives). There is a natural tendency to give the most time to the patient (or relative) who is the most assertive in demanding or requesting that time. But a policy of dividing one's time according to demand is clearly unjust, for less assertive or demanding patients may benefit more from professional time, and may be more seriously harmed by being allocated insufficient time. Similarly, it will always be necessary to discriminate between patients who would benefit from care in a specialist unit, such as the coronary care unit, intensive unit, or specialist palliative care unit. There will always be more patients who would benefit from such specialist care than there are places in those units. Decisions here cannot mechanically follow 'guidelines'; qualitative judgements are required, and those making them must be prepared to take responsibility for them.

Even when morally justifiable methods of discrimination are used in micro-allocation the public, patients, and doctors all tend to feel very uncomfortable with the whole exercise and the results. There is general distress when a life-prolonging treatment, or one that would alleviate suffering, is denied to one patient in order to provide it to another, even when that other patient would derive greater benefit from it. Most distress and adverse media publicity usually occur when a patient is denied a life-prolonging treatment. This is partly because the consequences—possibly death—are so serious for the patient who does not receive the treatment. It might also be argued that everyone has an equal desire or interest in staying alive, and that since this characteristic is the same, then discrimination between them on any other grounds is not justifiable. But we have said that there is a moral requirement to maximize the health benefit from scarce resources, and so the net benefit expected from the rationed treatment must be a highly relevant characteristic or criterion in the rationing process.

The language used to describe the rationing of life-prolonging treatments, particularly in the media, tends to exacerbate emotional reactions to discrimination between individuals. Such treatments are usually described as 'life-saving', which leads to the notion that if society does not provide them it has *failed* to save a life. There is a strong general presumption of the rightness of trying to save lives in society, and it is generally considered a moral obligation to save a life if one can do so without risk to other lives. Therefore, the use of the term 'life-saving' to describe a treatment entails a moral obligation to provide the treatment, whereas the term 'life-prolonging' is not associated with the notion of a moral obligation.

It can, and should, be argued that the term 'life-saving' with regard to medical treatment is misleading in most cases. If a curative treatment for an otherwise terminal illness can be given to a child or young person, one might reasonably argue that such treatment 'saves' a life. But such treatments would be provided by a decent minimum of health care, unless they were extraordinarily expensive or themselves entailed severe suffering. In the context of resource allocation in health care it is important always to remember that ultimately all patients will die. For this reason it makes much more sense to speak of life-prolonging or life-sustaining treatments, rather than life-saving treatments —for no life can be 'saved' forever. Furthermore, most life-prolonging treatments actually extend life by only 10 or 20 years, not a whole average life-span. Thus it is misleading to imply that such treatments have 'saved' a whole life.

In discriminating between individuals there is general acceptance of the formal principle of justice previously mentioned— that equals should be treated equally, and unequals unequally. This means that people who are equal in all the relevant characteristics or criteria should be treated the same, whilst those who are different in relevant characteristics or criteria should be treated differently. The moral problem lies in deciding what are the relevant characteristics or criteria on which we should discriminate between patients in the process of micro-allocation.

The most obvious criterion, and one which is generally agreed to be morally justifiable, is what we might call *medical utility*, or the expectation of medical benefit from the treatment. Obviously, assessment of benefit must include assessment of the likelihood of benefit for each patient, as well as its magnitude. For example, if one kidney is available and there are two potential recipients, the likelihood of success of the transplant is as relevant as the length of time that the transplant might add to the life of each patient. If one patient is a diabetic the chances of success of the transplant in that patient are less, so if other clinical features are similar then the transplant should go to the non-diabetic patient. Arguments can be mounted for and against a list of other criteria for micro-allocation such as age, social utility, queuing, prior commitment, quality of life, or lottery.

In deciding which of these criteria are morally acceptable for decisions about who should or should not receive treatment, the clinician is involved in questions of evidence as it affects specific patients, and his own judgements of likely benefit. These decisions are painful and controversial, but from the point of view of this book, they illustrate the mixture of scientific evidence and humane judgement.

5.9 Clinical judgement and society

Those who dismiss clinical judgement are apt to see it as a matter for individuals—the clinician and his patient. But a consideration of the problems of just resource management brings out that evidence and judgement cannot be adequately analysed at an individualistic level. The judgements of clinicians, especially hospital clinicians, lead to the commitment of resources, mainly the taxpayers' resources. There is, therefore, an onus on clinicians—a moral responsibility—to act as trustees of these resources. In other words, evidence and judgement have a social dimension. This does not cast doubt on the Downie–Macnaughton thesis but rather extends it. The evidence-base of treatments must include all the costs—including continuing care in the community —and the clinical judgement must be tempered by the knowledge that all patients share a right to equal consideration.

5.10 Conclusions

1. There is overwhelming evidence, deriving from considerations of finance and equity, that health care rationing is necessary.
2. Doctors' objections to rationing are based on misunderstandings; they are trustees of resources.
3. Macro-allocation cannot be based on the QALY, but requires judgement about the characteristics of the population, about treatment and care, and the use of relevant moral principles.
4. Micro-allocation is unavoidable but unpleasant.
5. Various suggested criteria for micro-allocation have limited usefulness and cannot be an automatic substitute for the doctor's judgement.

6. Clinical judgement has a social dimension because doctors, especially hospital consultants, are trustees of resources.

References

1. Daniels N, The ideal advocate and limited resources. *Theoretical Medicine*, 1987; 8: 69–75.
2. Culyer AJ, The rationing debate. Maximising the health of the whole community: the case for. *BMJ* 1997; 314: 667–9.
3. Beauchamp TL, Childress JF, *Principles of Biomedical Ethics* (4th edn). Oxford, Oxford University Press, 1994.
4. Edgar A, Salek S, Shickle D, Cohen D, *The Ethical QALY*. Haslemere, UK, Euromed Communications, 1998, p.4.
5. Edgar *et al.* op. cit.
6. Downie RS, The value and quality of life. *Journal of the Royal College of Physicians and Surgeons of London* 1999; 33: 378–81.
7. Aristotle *The Nicomachean Ethics* Trans D.Ross. Oxford: Oxford University Press, 1980, Book V.

6 Educating judgement: the humanities

6.1 Introduction

This book has so far attempted to describe the knowledge, skills, and attributes required for someone to make good clinical judgements. It is clear that the doctor needs to understand his patient through a scientific knowledge of how the body works and appreciate how scientific research can help him make decisions about how best to treat a patient. But we have also discussed the ways in which this evidence-base must be modified in the clinic; a 'humane' doctor is required with the understanding (the interpretative ability and insights), governed by ethical sensitivity, to apply, in the particular clinical situation, scientific evidence and skills. As we shall see, a broad education is also required. This chapter is concerned with providing more detail on this capacity for humane judgement, and with considering how far it can be learned. Before we embark on this we should note that little will be said here directly about education for scientific judgement. This is because it is a large and important topic on its own, with a large literature.

It is a lot to expect from the average student, who emerges from medical school at the age of 22 or 23, to start working as a house officer. It is also a lot to expect from the university, which has prepared them for this role. In fact, we might raise the question as to why medicine is a subject that is studied at university at all. Medicine can be seen as a very practical job, and the knowledge and skills required to practise can be attained primarily by apprenticeship. In this sense the process of becoming a doctor might be regarded as like that of becoming a plumber or a car mechanic. There is a certain amount of factual information to be learned but most of the job is learned at the side of someone who is already skilled at it. However, in Chapters 2–3, we suggested that there is more to the job of being a doctor than knowledge and skills. Is this extra dimension also to be acquired by apprenticeship, and if not, how can we make sense of the process of developing young people as doctors in educational terms?

We have described the attitude that enables the good doctor to reach sound judgements as a 'humane' attitude. Now, many writers on medical ethics would gloss this as an *ethically* sensitive attitude, and take the view that what the good doctor needs, in addition to technical competence, is a capacity for ethics. This is certainly important, and we shall begin by saying something about it (Section 6.2). But, as we have already suggested in Chapter 3, the concept of the humane doctor is wider than that of the ethical doctor. The humane doctor has an educational breadth, as well as an ethical sensitivity. We shall go on to develop the idea of the educated doctor as an introduction to the broader idea of the humane doctor (Section 6.3). It will emerge that the humane doctor who can exercise insightful judgement, is both broadly educated and ethically sensitive.

6.2 Teaching ethics

As we have seen, the doctor has evidence-based knowledge and skills, and applies them in a humane manner in the clinic. As we said at the beginning of the chapter, the problem of how best to teach this knowledge and skills is a large topic on its own. Medical schools have been experimenting world-wide on 'problem-based learning' and other methods. The jury is still out on these experiments, and we shall not here enter into these debates. Just as difficult is the question of whether, and if so how, humane attitudes can be taught and, if they can be taught, what room there can be in the curriculum for such teaching, and how it can be integrated with the aims and objectives of medical education. These are the questions that will concern us in the next few sections of this chapter.

There can be some concerns, as we have said, about whether the teaching of morality and attitudes to medical students is successful or even possible. It may be that the only way some students will learn such things is by experiencing more of life for themselves. However, the reality is that those of us who are involved in the education of future doctors have an obligation both to the students, to prepare them for the problems they will encounter, and to their future patients, who need to be protected against the insensitivities of the young. The GMC lists 12 'attitudinal objectives' in *Tomorrow's Doctors*[1] and these include:

(1) respect for patients and colleagues that encompasses, without prejudice, diversity of background and opportunity, language, culture, and way of life;

(2) awareness of the moral and ethical responsibilities involved in individual patient care and in the provision of care to populations of patients; such awareness must be developed early in the course.

Hence, teaching morality or ethics is a curriculum requirement.

We will discuss four methods of raising awareness of attitudes and of moral issues. They are not, of course, exhaustive or exclusive, and indeed the employment of a combination of them would be desirable. As an introduction, however, we shall consider the logically prior idea of the morally good doctor.

6.2.1 The morally good doctor

There is an element of the logically odd in the idea of the morally good doctor, which can be brought out if we compare it with the idea of the morally good plumber or the morally good airline pilot.[2] In the (highly unlikely) circumstance of someone saying, 'Mr X is a morally good airline pilot', we might judge that two claims had been run together: 'Mr X is an airline pilot' and 'Mr X is morally good'. These two claims do not have much to do with each other, and are oddly yoked together in that we tend to appraise morally and appraise technically in different types of context. Thus it would be perfectly possible for someone to be a pilot (or a plumber, or a musician, or a systems analyst, or a gardener) and not be morally good. It is even possible for someone to be a *good* pilot, plumber, musician, systems analyst, gardener, and not be morally good. For in these cases, the occupational names refer to the technical skills or sets of skills that define a given occupation, whereas the term 'morally good' refers to the character of the person who happens to have the skills. Moreover, the technician may even exercise the skills for a bad end. For example, let us imagine a good (i.e. highly skilled) computer operator who is not only morally bad, in that he exploits his employees, beats his wife, etc., but also uses his computer skills to hack into confidential files about patients, which he proceeds to sell to insurance companies. Thus we can say of some skilled persons (i.e. a good pilot, builder, etc.) that (1) personally they are bad, and (2) that they may sometimes use their skills for a bad end.

Can the same be said of the doctor? Plato certainly thought so. He is quite explicit that the good doctor can be a good poisoner. He adopts this position because, in common with other Greek thinkers, he classifies medicine as a *techne,* a craft comparable to that of the carpenter or ship's captain. For Plato, the 'good doctor' is 'good at' something: moral goodness in our sense does not come into it.[3] Indeed, the Hippocratic Oath, which requires the physician to work for the benefit of, and not to harm, patients, is probably not concerned with 'beneficence' and 'non-maleficence' in the modern sense. The Hippocratic Oath refers to the 'art' (i.e. 'craft') of medicine and is concerned that the craftsman (the physician) should not attempt to do what his skills do not enable him to do to his materials (patients). In terms of this approach, the good doctor will certainly have virtues, but they will be the virtues of the good craftsman rather than moral virtues in our modern sense. To teach someone to be a good doctor would, therefore, be to teach a complex craft. Plato does, of course, discuss the question of whether moral virtue can be taught, but he does not think that moral virtue is a *techne.* If we agree with Plato, then we are agreeing that the phrase 'morally good doctor' is odd because of the juxtaposition of technical excellence and moral excellence in the one phrase. But is Plato right in seeing the practice of medicine as just a *techne* or, more accurately, should we in the modern world think of medicine as just a set of skills? Are there any special moral qualities that are needed by the doctor *qua* doctor?

The dominant fashion in medical ethics for the last 20 years has been to assert that a doctor requires the following moral qualities: a desire to avoid harming the patient (non-maleficence), a desire to help (beneficence), a desire to act justly, and a desire to respect the patient's autonomous decisions. The trouble with these 'four principles' is not that they are irrelevant to the life of a doctor: it is that they are relevant to any occupation because they are among the basic principles governing harmonious and co-operative social life. There is nothing specific and essential to medicine about them. Are there any moral qualities that are specific to, or at least integral to, the practice of medicine?

To find these we must first look at what doctors actually do, and what they do is intimately connected with the needs of patients (Section 3.5). Typically, patients will have an illness, disease, injury, ailment (all of them real or imagined), or will require advice on diet, contraception, or future lifestyle. As a result of their real or imaginary conditions, patients will feel vulnerable, confused, insecure, powerless, hopeless, aggressive, despondent, and so on. To respond well to patients who may exhibit a range of these characteristics, a doctor will need to be humane and compassionate, to be imaginative, in the sense of being able to see the problem from the patient's perspective, and to convey calmness and equanimity. Other occupations may also need such qualities, but they are integral to the practice of medicine. In other words, the practice of medicine is not simply the exercise of a technical skill, because moral qualities are built into it. It will follow that the oddness of the phrase 'morally good doctor' is not that of an incongruous yoking together, but that of verbal redundancy.

The position we have reached is sufficiently complex to require restatement. We began by drawing attention to the fact that the expression 'morally good doctor' is logically odd. If we construe the oddness in terms of an analogy with 'morally good carpenter' it will consist in the running together of two distinct modes of appraisal—the technical and the moral. If the practice of medicine were simply the exercise of a *techne* or set of skills, we would have correctly identified the source of the oddness. But medicine is more than a *techne*. Certain moral virtues (not the 'four principles') are intimately bound up with the practice of medicine: the good doctor must have at least some moral virtues. In other words, at least some qualities of the morally good person, such as compassion, imagination, and equanimity, must be built into the concept of the good doctor. Because of the nature of the material on which the doctor works—human beings—the art of medicine must be more than simply a technique. To put it another way, the concept of a doctor is not morally neutral, as that of 'carpenter' or 'pilot' might be; it is evaluative. Hence the oddness of the phrase 'morally good doctor' is the oddness of pleonasm; for doctors to be morally good is for them to act as good doctors. This is not to say that doctors must have every moral virtue, but only that good medical practice must be humane and governed by practical wisdom. We hope, of course, that the doctor also acts in terms of the 'four principles', but then we *all* should, for they are amongst the principles of good citizenship, rather than anything especially to do with medicine.

6.2.2 Methods of teaching medical ethics

We shall not discuss methods in detail here, for there is a large literature,[4,5,6,7,8] but simply mention four methods that can be used in conjunction. The first is the most traditional and consists of a lecture, often given by a moral philosopher, on basic theories of moral philosophy. Unless this is done well it can easily seem remote and abstract to medical students, although it can be much more successful with practising doctors who have already experienced problems for themselves in the clinic. The initial impetus to the health-care ethics movement came from a fusion of medical concerns with moral philosophy, and that is still the main source of energy. When moral philosophy dominates, however, the discussion can easily become too abstract. The reason is that philosophers tend to use fanciful examples to test the edges of concepts, but when this practice is carried over into the teaching of medical ethics, it can seem alien to medical realism. One antidote to abstraction is to use case-histories.

This is the second and most common method of teaching ethics. It appeals to students because actual cases can be used and this creates the atmosphere of realism, which is essential if medicine, nursing, or other health-care students are to treat the subject seriously. Certainly it is important that cases should be related to general principles and broad lessons drawn from such discussion, but without the clinical details students will lose interest.

Reservations about the 'case-history approach' to the teaching of medical ethics have been expressed by Coope.[9] He makes three points: that case histories can suggest that moral decision-making is harder than it really is; that factual details can obscure the moral features (if any) in a case; and that the very consideration of some sorts of cases can be corrupting or desensitizing. There is something of merit in all three points, although the criticisms are robustly (perhaps too robustly) rejected by Gillon,[10] for all that is really being advocated by Coope is care and realism in the case-histories that are chosen. Clearly, case-histories have an important role to play if they are seen as 'triggers' to discussion and as stimuli for thought. They are essentially 'coat-pegs' on which to hang concepts and views. We shall not discuss them further, since their effectiveness is widely known.

A third method of teaching ethics is the use of a diary. Students are encouraged to record problems they may encounter in their clinical work, or which they note in the work of others. This again is effective in that it relates ethics to the student's own experiences.

A fourth method is the use of the arts. This is now being widely recommended. What can medical students learn from the arts? We have argued elsewhere[11] that literature and drama gives rise to moral questions and also develop our capacities to answer them. It is tempting to follow the philosophers and think of the resolution of moral questions in terms of the application of principles supported by rational argument. Principles and logic certainly have their place, but the arts can extend our imagination and deepen our sympathies, and these capacities are also essential to the wise, humane, and caring doctor. The point here is that philosophers, like biological and social scientists, must stand back from the phenomena and present their accounts in detached prose style. On the other hand, the arts involve us directly and make us vividly and emotionally aware of what it is like to be in the situation that the philosopher and social scientist discuss, of what it means to be ill oneself, or to be a relative or helper of someone who is ill. In this way the arts develop compassion. Moreover, the arts can provide a cognitive shaping to emotion. There is a danger that those in the caring professions develop a generalized attitude of caring. The arts can help us develop what we shall call compassion-in-the-particular-situation.

We have already maintained (Section 2.7) that communication skills are of importance to the good doctor. It can be argued[12] that this is one area to which the arts can make a major contribution. For example, literature focuses attention on language, on the connotations and resonances of words used to describe or express feelings and fears. There is a two-way process here. We tend to concentrate on the doctor's communication with the patient, because it is for failures there that doctors are often criticized. A study of the many ways in which literary writers communicate with their readers can be of help here. But patients also try to communicate, and awareness of the nature of the anecdote (Section 2.4) can help doctors to understand what patients are telling them and how patients perceive their illnesses.[13]

Painting brings out the non-verbal ways in which feelings or attitudes can be expressed. Consider, for example, the sympathetic portrayal of the doctor in the painting *The Doctor* by Sir Luke Fildes,[14] which hangs in the Tate Gallery in London. The main features of this painting (from the medical point of view) are the curve of the doctor's back as he leans forward, the concentration of his gaze, and the shadowy figure of the anxious parents behind the sick child's bed. As an illustration of the doctor–patient relationship, this has an eloquent sensitivity that communicates itself more directly than a treatise. No amount of science or philosophy can succeed in conveying, with the subtlety and infinite variety of the arts, this basic aspect of human relationships and, therefore, of doctor–patient relationships.

Teaching communication skills can be seen as a technique, simply a morally neutral skill. But if it is taught via the arts, it is embedded into a moral framework. The student learns by imaginative identification with the situation depicted in the art.

These then are four methods of teaching morality. There are others, such as role-play, but they are all compatible and some combination would be desirable. It is to be hoped that these methods and others will raise the ethical consciousness of medical students. But ethical sensitivity is only one of the two components in the humane attitude. We shall now move on to consider the other aspect of the humane attitude.

The second main component of the humane attitude—which reveals itself, as does ethical sensitivity, in humane judgements—is educatedness in various aspects. We shall now turn to a discussion of this.

6.3 Education and training

How is it that medical schools attract the highest achievers in secondary schools but those who have gone through the experience of medical education do not regard themselves as educated? Part of the answer to this question lies in the poor state of medical education in recent years and the disappointment many aspiring doctors feel at the experience they have had at university as intelligent young people. But there is another way in which this question can be answered. Doctors who consider themselves not 'educated' may still feel that they are competent practitioners and well able to do the job that their university studies prepared them to do. We may say, then, that they might consider themselves as 'trained' doctors. Let us now consider the distinction between these two concepts of education and training, since the distinction is the key to the idea of the humane. These distinctions are based on the writings of the philosopher of education, RS Peters.[15,16]

Both education and training may be regarded as processes through which an individual must pass in order to become educated or trained. However, we do not tend to speak of a particular end or subject matter when we refer to education, as in 'I was educated in art or physiology': this sounds strange to us. But when we talk of someone as being 'trained', the immediate questions are, 'In what?', 'To do what?', or 'For what?'[17] Training implies preparation for carrying out a particular task or learning a specific skill. Medical students might be trained to take blood from patients or to examine the heart correctly. Such activities involve a narrow focus on the task and practice in order to develop the ability to carry it out. In contrast, we never speak of a person being 'educated' for a specific end. 'Education' is connected with '*educere*' = 'to lead out' and implies a broadening and widening of the vision and the mind. The first distinction, then, between education and training is that training necessarily involves a narrowing of the focus to concentrate on learning a specific task or skill, whereas education has to do with opening out, with releasing and liberating.[18]

The second point, which distinguishes education from training, is that educational processes must have what Peters calls a wide 'cognitive perspective'.[19] Subjects such as science, literature, and history are regarded as valuable educationally because knowledge of these subjects contributes to knowledge and understanding in many other areas. For example, we would be surprised to hear a scholar of Dickens speak only of the fact that Dickens' books are good stories, without referring to the social comment and social history they contain. In the same way, the botanical process of apoptosis, which describes the 'falling away' of leaves from the trees in autumn, has been used by medical scientists in cancer research to stimulate an understanding of a similar process in cells.

In other words, it is not a sufficient condition of being educated that someone has had a training in science or history. It is possible to be a scientist or a historian without seeing the connections with other disciplines or the wider world, although such scientists or historians may not be very effective. The ability to make connections and be excited by such connections between one discipline and another reflects a certain attitude of mind: an attitude that we would associate with the humanely educated person. This is Adam Smith's point (see Section 1.6) to which we can now return: 'Philosophy is the science of the connecting principles of nature'. This attitude of mind is reflected in the idea that education is of the whole person, not just one part of the mind or body, as in training; and it is characterized by openness to ideas and experiences, and a willingness to change in response to these ideas and experiences.

It is difficult to contemplate how such an attitude of mind can be encouraged by the educational process. It might be argued that this openness is present in some students and not in others and that it cannot be put there if it is not there already. This is a particular problem in the context of vocational courses like medicine because students tend to regard as valuable only those classes which they see as directly relevant to the job of being a doctor. Medical students have traditionally looked down on subjects such as psychology or sociology which they see as being at best common sense and at worst unimportant to their future clinical work.

Peters' third point about an educational process is related to the second. We have characterized the educated person as someone who is open to new ideas and who is able to see connections and make links between different disciplines. It follows from this that such a person must be open to being changed by these new thoughts and ideas or, to use Peters' terminology, his whole 'outlook may be transformed'. It is possible for a person to be trained as a car mechanic or a cook and not be changed by the experience. The knowledge they have gained remains external to themselves as persons, and can be lifted and laid when required. In contrast, an educational process involves the whole person and the knowledge they acquire becomes integral to them and cannot be laid aside; rather it affects other thoughts and experiences they have, and may unexpectedly bring about new ideas when they are focusing on an apparently unrelated subject.

We can say, therefore, that an educational process should bring about change in its subject. Peters takes this further, in a fourth point about education, by saying that the change should be for the better, not the worse.[20] In other words, something valuable or worthwhile for its own sake must be passed on by any process regarded as education. This point may seem to make any discussion about whether the process of learning medicine should properly be called education a pointless one, as medicine is clearly a worthwhile thing to do. However, Peters' point is related to the value of the knowledge and the subject *in itself*, rather than on what it equips the student to do. In medicine, the study of things like human biology, psychology, and sociology, may be regarded as intrinsically valuable, as these subjects provide ways of making sense of the world and widening the student's understanding of it. A degree in arts does not equip students for any particular job but those who ask arts students, 'What is your degree for?' are entirely missing the point. The point of doing it is purely for the experience of studying subjects that will broaden the mind and widen the outlook in a valuable way.

Part of a degree in medicine involves learning things that cannot be regarded as intrinsically valuable or as making a change in the person who learns them. The knowledge of how to take blood from a patient is only of extrinsic value, as assisting in patient care, and in no other way. Repeating the act many times may make the students more skilled and dextrous but it will make no change in them cognitively. This is not to say that being trained in this skill is not important; education and training must go hand in hand in learning medicine.

It follows from this fourth point about education that if the educational process should aim to bring about a positive change in someone through the study of something worthwhile, then the person engaged in the process should be interested in, and come to care about, what they are doing.[21] It would be difficult to call someone educated who had been through a degree in English literature and after graduating never picked up a novel or read a poem again. Education is not a process that ends after school or university is finished. As Peters expresses it:

...to be educated is not to have arrived; it is to travel with a different view.[22]

Fifth, if the educated person is to care about his subject and to allow it to change his outlook, the educator must adopt person-respecting methods in his educational approach. Learning by coercion, indoctrination, or repetition, cannot be called education because it will not involve understanding or widening of the person's perspective, as we have described. Knowledge gained in this way will tend to be 'inert'[23] with no possibility of change or development. Training can involve processes such as coercion, imitation, and repetition.[24] A surgeon who wishes to be trained in laparoscopic surgery must begin by copying his superior's

technique and then developing his own by repeating the operation many times. It would be perfectly legitimate in this training
process for the teacher to insist that the trainee surgeon performed the operation in a certain way, if this was the safest and
easiest way to get the best results. But this could not count as an
educational process.

In summary, then, we can say that an educational process
must lead to an opening out and a broadening of the educated
person's perspective, and what is learnt should have intrinsic
value. The educated person should be open to being changed by
the process, and that change should be positive and valuable.
In contrast, training may require a narrowing of the focus to
concentrate on learning a specific task, and there is no
expectation that the trained person will be changed by this
process or that he will think differently about the world as a
result. Rote learning, imitation, and even coercion, may be useful
techniques for training, but these have no place in the process of
education.

Where does the process of learning medicine fit in with these
ideas on training and education?[25] We might want to suggest
that, as medicine is a vocational course whose aim is to produce
people who can work as doctors at the time when they complete
the course, it is primarily a training process. This conclusion
might seem, in the light of our first point about the distinction
between education and training, to have some validity. In
contrast to students who graduate with arts degrees, for students
who have taken a degree in medicine it is quite clear what their
course is *for*, and we might describe them as 'trained' to be
doctors. Inasmuch as the medical degree has this narrow focus of
preparing students to be doctors it might again be more
appropriately termed a training activity rather than an educational one. However, this is an oversimplified account and can be
criticized in three ways.

First, educational as well as training activities take place
within the context of a medical degree. Students may be trained
in the skills of clinical examination by copying an experienced
clinician but they also take courses in which they learn about
biochemistry, physiology, and human anatomy. These courses
can be taught in a way that encourages a broad understanding of

the human body and its functions in the normal state—
understanding that is valuable for its own sake and can be the
focus of continuing interest and study beyond graduation.

Second, one of the points about a training activity was that it
has a narrow focus that prepares the trainee for a defined task. It
would be very difficult to describe the task of the doctor in this
way. Medicine comprises many jobs and requires adaptability in
its practitioners. Rightly or wrongly (see Section 3.5), patients
expectations of their doctors are wide and spread beyond the
confines of any narrowly defined clinical training. It would be
inappropriate, therefore, to describe the process of preparing
students for the job of being doctors as having a narrow focus.

The third criticism of our initial description of medicine as a
training involves a challenge to the distinctions made by Peters
between education and training. These distinctions need not be
as exclusive as has been suggested. The account given above
assumes that an educational process aims at the growth of
understanding (an aim intrinsic to the activity) and that a
training process aims at gaining some skill, which will make no
difference to the understanding the trainee has about what he is
engaged in (an aim extrinsic to the activity). However, this may
not be the case in all situations. It may be that in order for an
educational aim to be achieved (i.e. for understanding to be
advanced), the student needs to achieve a training aim first. An
example here might be that, for a student fully to understand the
three-dimensional anatomy of a woman's pelvis, he or she must
first learn the skill of pelvic examination.

In conclusion, then, preparing students to become doctors is
both an educational and a training activity. In that both these
processes are involved, and that medicine has a broad focus, it is
a legitimate concern of universities. We can, therefore, add
educatedness to ethical sensitivity as the second component in
the humane attitude.

6.4 Medical ethos

Before making a suggestion about how the second component in
the humane attitude—educatedness—might be cultivated, we

shall outline the nature of the unconscious resistance within medicine to such a development. It derives from what we shall call, following Downie and Charlton, the medical 'ethos'.[26] We shall summarize their argument.

The medical ethos is a practical one, in that it is directed towards action. This would seem to derive from the constraints of clinical practice, in which a decision must always be made, even if that decision is to postpone the decision.

This shows in the medical view of science. As we have argued (Section 1.7), for a doctor, science is a goal-directed activity, and the direction is towards improved clinical practice. In contrast, the scientist is regulated by goals *internal* to science itself (this is what is meant by science 'for its own sake'). It also shows in medical impatience with speculation of all kinds: indeed a 'short attention span', sometimes showing itself as a hard-headed approach, is often a fault of clinicians—although it is a 'fault' that has the benefits of efficiency and productivity in clinical practice.

The authors point out that 'decision' is a key word, because it is also characteristic of doctors to be decisive. When the caricature doctor is at fault, it is more often for deciding too soon (without sufficient consideration of evidence) than too late: at any rate, doctors do not usually experience much psychological difficulty about making up their minds. Such resolution contrasts with the attitudes of some other professions—and is one explanation of why doctors tend to adopt a dominant role on committees! Again, medicine is characterized by a high level of collegiality or solidarity. This is a great source of strength, as well as a possible source of harm, as when in the face of any criticism there is a tendency for doctors always to stick together. Downie and Charlton then proceed to examine how medical education is involved in the process of producing the medical ethos.

One part is the evolution of an *esprit de corps*. Various factors combine to produce *esprit de corps* within the medical school. First, the students are divided into classes (often large) each of which is treated as a unit, and the classes are all taught together in big lecture and practical sessions, whenever this is possible. Furthermore, all the students in the same class share a curriculum that is broadly, and sometimes exactly, the same as those of other class members. Such features are common to many medical schools during the preclinical period. The sheer bulk of information may forcibly impose the subject on the minds of the undergraduates. To some extent the medical students are usually physically set apart from other under-graduates in a medical school or college. And, commonly, curricular activities are reinforced by informal students' societies. Such factors may play a greater or lesser role in inculcating a sense of loyalty, tradition, or whatever it might be called, even in the earliest years; an attitude that becomes directed partly at the institution and its members, but also towards medicine itself.

In the clinical years, the process gathers momentum; the university terms are longer and vacations shorter; a standard of quasi-professional behaviour and dress is encouraged; 'out of hours' study is increasingly expected. Some factors are estab-lished explicitly, by lecture or textbook; but most of the medical ethos comes from apprenticeship, from the learning process described as 'modelling', whereby the acolyte becomes identified with the 'master' across a whole range of interlinking behaviour, attitudes, and emotions. This is the time during which the beginnings of a 'bedside manner' are adopted, and ways of relating to patients, other health-care workers and the public are internalized. This induction may be very enjoyable; and it is usual that the clinical years at medical school are the time of the greatest idealism concerning the values of a medical way of life.

Downie and Charlton point out that the fact of professional solidarity is a double-edged weapon, but its benefits should not be underestimated. In the first place, medicine is intrinsically an unpleasant job, in the sense that it involves contact with blood, sweat, and tears (and worse); but, more seriously, it involves life-and-death decisions and actions. All of which means that a mistake may have consequences of the utmost seriousness—and everybody makes mistakes. It is of the greatest importance that, on the one hand, mistakes can be acknowledged and corrected, and on the other hand, that the junior doctor is supported through the mistakes to develop the highest level of skill (because if 'everybody makes mistakes', then this applies particularly to the inexperienced new recruit).

The important point for our argument is that the medical ethos is not the whole story because it is inevitably incomplete. It is concerned only with certain limited aspects of life—with illness and disease. Medical solidarity can allow medicine to overstep its bounds—it can lead to a lack of perspective. If medicine is to function properly it must be placed within the scheme of society as a whole—its limits defined, its relationship to other world-views made clear. It is not satisfactory that the medical viewpoint should simply take over all other viewpoints by default, that the problems of life should all be medicalized. So that while the existence of what we have called medical ethos is important, we must also emphasize that this will be a good thing only if it is taken in perspective. Doctors, through a combination of excessive busyness and solidarity, can easily lose their broad perspectives to become, not just workaholic, but blinkered to the point of not knowing *when* to use their medical skill—although they might know very well *how*. This is often said to be the characteristic sin of the surgeon—yet it applies across a much wider spread of the profession. Hence it is important for the humane doctor to have, not only ethical sensitivity, but a broad perspective on life. This is necessary to ensure humane judgement.

6.5 Broadening the ethos

Granted this resistance to a broad humane outlook in medicine, how, if at all, can we teach medical students and anyone else in the health-care professions to acquire the humane qualities necessary for excellence in the practice of the professions? Or how can we broaden the ethos? One suggestion is that the practice of medicine can be humanized through the experience of what can be called a 'counter-culture'.[27]

In an academic sense, in medical education, this may mean exposing students to other disciplines in other academic contexts. Medical students often have the impression, and are encouraged in it by medical teachers, that they have an intellectual and moral superiority over other students. Perhaps it should be part of their education—it is in some universities—to be obliged to submit themselves to other disciplines. In the USA, for example, medicine is most often a postgraduate degree. This has two beneficial consequences: students are a little more mature when they begin their medical studies, and they have already been exposed to an academic counter-culture. We can even go beyond the purely academic and suggest that students should be encouraged to, and should be given curriculum space to, engage in activities that are not academic at all—sport, youth work, and so on. It is from this counter-culture, rather than from the exclusive study of medical ethics, that a sense of our common humanity may come.

6.6 The humane attitude: practicalities

It might be argued that even if our views on the 'counter-culture' have something to be said for them, they have no realistic hope of being adopted by medical faculties. Now this would have been true a few years ago, but an influential and authoritative document has changed all that. The new structure of the medical course, laid down by the GMC in their document *Tomorrow's Doctors*, [28] provides a golden opportunity for non-medical subjects to be introduced in some depth to medical students in the form of special study modules (SSMs). We describe the content of two such modules in the Appendix to this chapter, but here we will explain in general terms what modules are designed to achieve in the new curriculum structure.

Tomorrow's Doctors describes the SSMs in this way:[29]

They are no less important than the core curriculum but they focus not on the immediate requirements of the pre-registration year but on the long-term intellectual and attitudinal demands of a professional life that will constantly be challenged by growth of knowledge and change of circumstance....They will give scope for variation in educational style and content and will provide opportunity for experimentation in curriculum design...the overall consequence will be a widening of the outlets for the expression of individuality and the competitiveness of medical schools.

And in commenting on the proposed subject matter of the modules it says:[30]

...the modules offered will depend on the interests, resources and individual enthusiasms of medical school staff and to some extent on the wider range of opportunities within their universities. It will be anticipated that the majority of modules will be based on subjects directly related to medicine...but they need not be exclusively so. As medical research advances, it will inevitably become increasingly dependent on the ideas and techniques of other disciplines...it is hoped that the student of tomorrow may be drawn to some of these other disciplines and that opportunities to study, for example, a language or to undertake a project related to literature, or the history of medicine, may be offered.

The implication, then, is that as well as contributing to the process of making a doctor, the modules should be a source of intellectual challenge for the students, harnessing their individual interests and enthusiasms.

The GMC's recommendations are timely. A survey of the hopes and concerns of a class of first-year entrants to medical school[31] has identified 'self-fulfilment' and 'personal challenge and variety' as their second most important hope (after the desire to help patients). Their most important concern (after family and personal relationships) related to a 'loss of self'; in particular there was a fear of becoming 'isolated' about 'issues outside medicine'. Medical schools are fortunate in that they attract intelligent and well-motivated students, but these students often have interests that lie outside the narrowly scientific and medical content of the core. The SSMs clearly have a role in stimulating these individual interests, and preserving and developing the sense of 'self' and of self-awareness that is essential to sympathetic doctoring.

6.6.1 Three categories of SSM

The GMC in *Tomorrow's Doctors* stress that SSMs should not deal entirely with medical subject matter, although most of them will, and they appear to identify three different types of SSM: the medical; the ancillary medical; and the non medical. It is important to stress that there are three different types of SSM, since, with the narrowing of the compulsory part of the curriculum within the core, the SSMs might become merely a repository for all the medical subjects that have been ejected. The GMC make the point that medicine cannot exist in a vacuum and that it is becoming increasingly important that students have some understanding of other disciplines on which medicine is increasingly coming to rely, e.g. mathematics, physics, and computing. SSMs with this kind of subject matter we might call 'ancillary medical' SSMs, as they have a non-medical subject matter but are directly relevant to the practice of medicine. A further distinction should be made between these first two types of SSM (the purely medical and the ancillary medical) and a third type, the 'non-medical'. *Tomorrow's Doctors* suggested that students might study a language, literature, or history. This is a radical suggestion, as medical students have never before been given time within the curriculum to study subjects with no direct relevance to medicine. We wish to explore in more detail the justification for the inclusion of these different types of SSMs in the new style curriculum, concentrating in particular on the ancillary medical and non medical options.

Medical SSMs

The inclusion of purely medical SSMs is easy to justify. In a crowded curriculum (even after pruning) it is impossible to include every medical subject area relevant to the experience of doctors. Here is an opportunity for students to pursue their own medical interests and for medical schools to demonstrate their strengths. For instance, not every medical school will have experts on tropical medicine able to offer a course to students. The medical SSMs, therefore, provide a chance for specialized work at the undergraduate level.

It is important to stress, however, that to make the SSMs merely a series of clinical clerkships in minor medical specialities, would be to defeat the purpose of radical curriculum change. The SSMs may indeed provide students with the opportunity to study in more detail a medical subject not included in the core but this period of study should differ from their mainstream clinical teaching in such a way that the learning process has not purely been one of osmosis but also of personal discovery (Section 6.3).

Ancillary medical SSMs

Tomorrow's Doctors makes a case for what we have called ancillary medical subjects, such as mathematics, physics, the social sciences, and philosophy, on the basis that the 'ideas and techniques' of these disciplines are increasingly informing the development of medicine. It is in this context that the concept of transferable skills can be introduced. Transferable skills are those that are learned in a non-medical context and then are transferred to be used in a medical situation. This concept has been discussed in relation to thinking-skills courses by Professor NC Boreham.[32] He expresses some doubt about whether a skill learned in one context can be transferred to another, particularly if the skill has been learned in a 'classroom' context and is to be used in a practical situation. However, if the skill learned is the *same* skill, then this is surely possible. An example of this might be computing skills. There might also be ancillary courses—often seen in the context of business and industry—where students learn about working in a team. The advantage of learning these skills in a context outwith medicine is that students can more easily focus on the particular skill they wish to acquire without worrying about such things as their lack of knowledge in front of patients. We will discuss the acquisition of the skill of analysis of argument in the context of an SSM in philosophy in the Appendix. There are, therefore, a wide range of ancillary subjects that might contribute to the training of doctors, and the choice depends on the interests and ingenuity of the particular medical school and its university.

Non-medical SSMs

Third, let us turn to the non-medical subjects. In general terms, the GMC sees SSMs as fulfilling an educational aim in as much as the students undertaking them will study a subject in depth and that it will be a subject that excites their interest and which they will research personally. This certainly applies to non-medical SSMs. However, learning medicine is also a training exercise[33] and even non-medical subjects can provide training in skills that are relevant to the practice of medicine. In addition,

non-medical subjects can help develop the human qualities
essential in a good doctor; and involvement with other
disciplines can help medical students avoid the insularity that
characterizes medical classes. We wish now to discuss in more
detail the four areas where non-medical subjects might make a
contribution to the development of future doctors: education,
training, development of personal qualities, and broadening
social contacts. It will become clear how these are elements in the
second component of the humane attitude—a broad education—
and as such will influence the doctor's humane judgements.

6.7 The humane attitude: components

6.7.1 Education

Someone with a humane attitude, who will be able to make
humane judgements, must be broadly educated. As we have
discussed in Section 6.3, an educational activity should satisfy
certain criteria: it should be worthwhile and valuable for its own
sake; it should have a wide cognitive perspective; it should
stimulate interest and dedication in the student; and it should
transform his outlook. A course in philosophy, for example, will
allow the student a chance to read some of the great thinkers and
help him to understand different ways of looking at the world.
A course in medical history can put present medical discoveries
in perspective and give the student some insight into the fact that
medical knowledge is not set in stone; a strong impetus for
continuing his education through life. Such courses will give
students the opportunity to stand outside their more narrowly
focused medical activities and look on them from a different
viewpoint, thus encouraging a critical and questioning attitude.
Medical schools are ideally situated to institute such courses as
they are, for the most part, within universities where experts in
many disciplines are on hand.

6.7.2 Adaptability: training and transferable skills

Non-medical subjects can provide training in skills that are
useful in a medical context, and in learning to transfer such skills

for use in medical practice, the student can learn adaptability. We have already introduced the idea of transferable skills and it can be used once again to justify the training potential of non-medical subjects. One example here might be a course in media studies. Here the student might be expected to learn about interviewing people and to use this skill in the context of interviewing patients. The role of the medical interviewer is the same as that of the journalist, in that both are trying to get at the truth of the situation. They differ in that the journalist aims purely to present the information to an audience, whereas the doctor aims to use the information to make a diagnosis and decide on treatment. However, medical students can learn from the journalist's investigative approach, the importance of focusing entirely on what the patient is saying. In the non-medical context this can be practised without, at the same time, being distracted by giving the patient an answer. A subject like philosophy (which also fulfils the educational criteria) can teach students to order thoughts, construct an argument, and reach a logical conclusion. These skills are essential in diagnosis, where the doctor must gather information to support a thesis and go through logical steps to reach a conclusion. This is an important consideration in medical training.

6.7.3 Personal development

We have seen that non-medical subjects should be allowed in SSMs because of their educational and training value. However, the practice of medicine is not just concerned with knowledge and skills but also with a humane and sympathetic approach to people. JS Mill in his essay *On Liberty* asserted:

It really is of importance, not only what men do, but also what manner of men they are that do it. Among the works of men, which human life is rightly employed in perfecting and beautifying, the first in importance surely is man himself.[34]

There has certainly not been much thought given to 'perfecting and beautifying' medical students through their educational process; rather that process has tended to brutalize and dehumanize.[35] It is here, perhaps, that a study of the arts, in the form of plays, poems, books, and paintings, can best be justified. Of course, studying the arts is also educational, in that it widens the understanding and has an intrinsic value. But in demanding an emotional response, the arts allow the reader or viewer to discover their own hidden values and prejudices, and to challenge them. In other words, the arts help students to develop self-awareness and enhance their understanding of the human condition. For young people, who emerge at the age of 22 or 23 to become doctors, the arts may provide some experience of life, albeit at second-hand, which is essential for their development as caring people.

One example of this potential of the arts to challenge values and beliefs would be in a study of the book *Trainspotting* by Irvine Welsh.[36] This book deals with the story of a young drug user and his friends, and is graphic in its descriptions of the process of 'shooting up', and uncompromising in its portrayal of the degradation that addiction brings. But in his use of humour and pathos, the author gives the addicts a human face. This book would force students to face up to their attitudes to drug users, so that they can recognize and overcome any feelings of fear or disgust, and help those who present to them as patients. So far in medicine it has been the role of ethics teaching to instruct students on their approach to patients but an understanding of ethical principles will not develop the sensitivities in the way that a study of the arts can.

6.7.3 Broadening the perspective: reducing insularity

Finally, in the course of studying non-medical subjects, students will have the opportunity of meeting people in other faculties. Medical classes tend to be rather insular because (as we have said), unlike in other faculties, the whole year follows the same curriculum. SSMs can provide some variety for students and allow them to show their unique interests. Having the chance to get to know teachers and students in other disciplines will help break this insularity, and may also, ultimately, foster better relationships between doctors and the outside world.

In conclusion, the introduction of SSMs to the curriculum has been proposed in order to improve the educational profile of medical schools. But in providing the chance to offer many subjects, not just medical, a new educational opportunity can be exploited. The neglected area of personal development can be more explicitly addressed through a study of the arts; and study in other disciplines will help future doctors appreciate the knowledge and skills of others.

6.8 Aims and objectives

6.8.1 Performance objectives

The standard educational approach, when creating new courses in medical schools at present, is to start by defining the course 'objectives'. The category of objective in use is the 'performance objective'. Performance objectives are behavioural indicators of the ways in which students will have changed by the end of a course.[37] Their advantages include communication of intent to prospective and actual students, and to other academics, the need to consider in detail the end-points or outcomes of teaching, and the provision of a basis for a systematic approach to course design, including assessment.

But not all useful learning is both predictable at the outset and demonstrable by the performance of some newly-learned skill.[38] An objectives-led approach also implies that the *outcome* of learning is the only important aspect, with the *process* being irrelevant. In the courses described in the appendix, dependence upon performance objectives can be seen as both restrictive and destructive. For example:

(1) it is likely that some changes that will occur in students, will not have been foreseen;[39]

(2) the precise direction of many of the changes is unpredictable, and dependent upon such factors as pre-existing individual knowledge, attitudes, and maturity;

(3) many changes will not be quantifiable and, therefore, not conducive to precise objective formulation; indeed, this may be true of any course in which the emphasis is on attaining knowledge and attitudes rather than skills, or where the aim is to educate rather than train.

These are some of the objections to objectives; others have been considered by Macdonald-Ross[40] and Eisner.[41] The latter moved to correct the imbalance caused by exclusive emphasis on 'performance objectives' by proposing the concept of 'expressive objectives'.

6.8.2 Expressive objectives

The focus of 'expressive objectives' is not on the student's ability to perform a task, but with less demonstrable changes like the development of skills and strategies in approaching problems, or appreciation of the ambiguities and interpretative problems of written or spoken language, or the ability to write a piece of clear and expressive English. 'Expressive objectives', therefore, are concerned with the process aspects of a course rather than the outcome.

Process-led approaches to higher education have been proposed by Stenhouse[42] and, more recently, by Laurillard.[43] Stenhouse generated a 'process model' for course design, which he describes as more appropriate than objectives models for areas that centre on knowledge and understanding. The aim of this model is to *develop* understanding, rather than to *gain* knowledge. This is done through inquiry and exploration, leading to 'induction into knowledge', which cannot be transferred but must come from within; students can be led to knowledge. Essentially, in this model, teaching then becomes a kind of extended conversation.[44]

This 'process model' has two important implications for this module. First, development of the teacher is inevitable alongside the development of the student. Teachers will learn both from the student and from the process of teaching. They can never teach the same way twice. This allows greater evolution, both for the teachers and for the course, than if the course were following a more prescriptive objectives-led model. Second, to use the language of social anthropology, the very process of learning can itself generate 'latent' outcomes, which may be more important than the 'manifest' outcomes.[45] For example, students might discuss a poem and come to understand that it is open to three interpretations. Knowledge of what these three interpretations are is the 'manifest' outcome of the discussion. But the 'latent' outcome is that students become aware that what patients say or do may be open to several interpretations. In other words, for a medical student, the importance of discussing a poem may derive from what they learn from the process of discussion itself, rather then from its outcome. If we take the analogy of someone going on a journey: their interest may be as much in what is learned on the journey as in the destination.

6.9 Humane judgement

Good clinical judgement involves a combination of technical judgement and humane judgement. In this chapter we have been examining the components of humane judgement and making some suggestions as to how they might be taught. Humane judgements, of course, flow from a humane attitude, and one obvious component of a humane attitude is ethical sensitivity. We stressed that there is more to ethical sensitivity than applying principles; virtues, such as equanimity, are involved. We suggested various methods by which ethical sensitivity might be developed.

The second main component in the humane attitude is educatedness, which we distinguished from being trained. There is a certain resistance in medicine to these broader ideas—a resistance that stems from the 'medical ethos'—and a 'counter-culture' is one possible antidote to this disabling ethos. The GMC has made possible a formal route by which a counter-culture might be established—by means of Special Study Modules.

In developing the idea of SSMs we were able to spell out the components of 'educatedness', which are relevant to the humane attitude. These are adaptability—in such matters as seeing logical connections—personal development, and the adoption of a broad perspective. In mounting courses to contribute to the cultivation of educatedness, we argued that 'expressive objectives' are more relevant than the conventional 'performance objectives'.

If the GMC's proposed revolution in medical education is to work, then the opportunities presented by SSMs must be grasped with both hands. We may, then, in 10 years time start producing doctors with a thirst to pursue their education throughout their lives and who are more rounded human beings.

6.10 Conclusions

1. There are problems concerning the nature of the 'humane attitude', and how to teach it.

2. The humane attitude has an ethical component and a broader educational component, which provides perspective.

3. The ethical component in the humane attitude can be taught via moral philosophy, case studies, keeping a diary, the arts, and any combination of these.

4. Education must be distinguished from training.

5. The 'ethos' of medicine is such that a 'counter-culture' is required, supplied by the study of the non-medical subjects, which provide the perspective.

6. The GMC has made the study of non-medical subjects possible by insisting on SSMs, which may be non-medical.

7. These may require 'expressive objectives' rather than 'performance objectives', for education is a 'process' and not just an 'outcome'.

References

1. General Medical Council, *Tomorrow's Doctors: Recommendations on Under-graduate Medical Education*. London: GMC, 1993, p.15.
2. Downie RS, Macnaughton RJ, Can we teach medical students to be morally good doctors? In *Advances in Bioethics* (ed. Evans M). Greenwich, Connecticut: JAI Press, 1998.
3. Plato, *Republic*. Trans. Lee D, second ed. Harmondsworth, Penguin, 1974, Book I, 332b–336a.
4. Boyd KM (ed.), *Report of a Working Party on the Teaching of Medical Ethics* (Chairman, Sir Desmond Pond). London: Institute of Medical Ethics Pub. Ltd., 1987.
5. Boyd KM, Teaching medical ethics to medical students and GP trainees. *Journal of Medical Ethics* 1987; 13: 132–3.
6. Gillon R, Thinking about a medical school core curriculum for medical ethics and law. *Journal of Medical Ethics* 1996; 22: 323–4.

7. Hope T, Ethics and law for medical students: the core curriculum. *Journal of Medical Ethics* 1998; 24: 147–8.
8. Consensus statement by teachers of medical ethics and law in UK medical schools. Teaching medical ethics and law within medical education: a model for the UK core curriculum. *Journal of Medical Ethics* 1998; 24: 188–92.
9. Coope CM, Teaching medical ethics: does teaching by cases mislead us about morality? *Journal of Medical Ethics* 1996; 22: 46–52.
10. Gillon R, Case studies and medical education. *Journal of Medical Ethics* 1996; 22: 2–4.
11. Downie RS, *The Healing Arts: an Illustrated Oxford Anthology*. Oxford: Oxford University Press 1994, p.xvi.
12. Downie, 1994, op. cit, p.xvi.
13. Macnaughton RJ, Anecdotes and empiricism. *BJGP* 1995; 45: 571–2.
14. Downie, 1994, op. cit, p.288.
15. Peters RS, *Ethics and Education*. London: George Allen and Unwin Ltd, 1966.
16. Peters RS (ed.), *The Concept of Education*. London: Routledge & Kegan Paul, 1967.
17. Peters, 1966, op cit, p.34.
18. Downie RS, Charlton B, *The Making of a Doctor*. Oxford: Oxford University Press, 1992, p.54.
19. Peters, 1966, op. cit, p.31.
20. Peters, 1966, op. cit, p.25.
21. Peters, 1966, op. cit, p.37.
22. Peters, 1967, op. cit, p.8.
23. Peters, 1967, op. cit, p.8.
24. Downie and Charlton, op cit, p.54.
25. Downie and Charlton, op. cit., pp.54–7.
26. Downie and Charlton, op. cit., pp.57–63.
27. Charlton B, Holistic medicine or the humane doctor? *BJGP* 1993; 43: 475–7.
28. GMC, op. cit., p.7.
29. GMC, op. cit., p.7.
30. GMC, op. cit., p.9.
31. Fields SA, Toffler WL, Hopes and concerns of a first year medical class. *Medical Education* 1988; 22: 488–91.
32. Boreham NC, The dangerous practice of thinking. *Medical Education* 1994; 28: 172–9.
33. Calman KC, Downie RS, Education and training in medicine. *Medical Education* 1988; 22: 488–91.
34. Mill JS, On Liberty (1859). In *Utilitarianism*. (ed. Warnock M). Glasgow: Collins, 1962, p.188.
35. Weatherall DJ, The inhumanity of medicine. *BMJ* 1994; 309: 1671–2.
36. Welsh I, *Trainspotting*. London: Martin, Secker and Warburg, 1993.
37. Romisowski AJ, *Designing Instructional Systems*. London: Kogan Page, 1981.
38. Downie RS, Hendry RA, Macnaughton RJ, Smith BH, Humanising medicine: a special study module. *Medical Education* 1997; 31: 276–80.
39. Stenhouse L, *An Introduction to Curriculum Research and Development*. London: Heinemann, 1975, p.92.
40. Macdonald-Ross M, Behavioural objectives: a critical review, in *Instructional Science 2*, 1–52. Amsterdam: Elservier Scientific Publishing Co., 1973.

41. Eisner D, Instructional and expressive objectives, in *Curriculum Design* Golby (ed. M, Greenwald J, West R). London: Croom Helm, 1969.
42. Stenhouse, op. cit., pp.85–97.
43. Laurillard D, *Rethinking University Teaching*. London: Routledge, 1993.
44. Pask G, Conversational techniques in the study and practice of education. *British Journal of Psychology* 1976; 46: 12–25.
45. Emmet D, *Function, Purpose and Powers*. London: Macmillan, 1958.

7 Conclusion: clinical judgement

The title of our book is *Clinical Judgement: Evidence in Practice*. We have examined the concepts in the title as they apply to medical research, to clinical practice, to public health, and to resource management.

The concept of evidence, as it is used by scientists, is logically related to that of an hypothesis. Information, data, observations, and experiments become 'evidence' when they are for or against a specific hypothesis. Moreover, the hypothesis concerns what is universally, or at least generally, believed to be the case. The concept of evidence as used by detectives or forensically differs in two respects: the data and observations *suggest* a hypothesis, rather than confirm or disconfirm one; and the hypothesis is about a particular or specific state of affairs, rather than one which is more generally the case. The concept of evidence that applies to *medical research* is like that of the scientist, and the concept that applies to *clinical consultations* is like that of the detective. The reason that the detective model of evidence is appropriate for the clinician is that he is dealing with *specific* patients. The relevant evidence for the clinician to establish diagnosis, prognosis, and treatment comes from or applies to *this* particular patient.

The sources of evidence in the clinic are, therefore, of different kinds. One important source is, of course, that obtained via scientific routes, with which a clinician should be familiar from the science elements in his training, from scientific papers, and from the advice of other scientifically minded clinicians. This kind of evidence must be adapted to suit a given patient from a given social environment. A second source of information about the diagnosis will be the patient's own stories or anecdotes. We can say either that anecdotes are not evidence, but rather are an alternative source of relevant information; or we can say that anecdotes are a kind of clinically relevant evidence. They are certainly of importance to the clinician.

In discussing science it emerged that judgement is an essential part of the scientist's activities. He must constantly consider the interpretation of X, whether it is really an example of Y or supports his conclusion, and what weight to place on certain factors or what relevance to give them. This was especially true of qualitative research and randomized trials. The same is true of the judgement of the detective. These are the technical or scientific manifestations of judgement, and they make up one of the two essential components of good clinical judgement.

In adapting the scientific evidence to the specific patient, and in making sense of the patient's anecdotes, the doctor is again involved in the process of interpretation. He may also have insights into the situation, which may lie behind the patient's presence in the surgery. For example, the clinician must interpret the patient's symptoms, listen to his anecdotes in case some clues emerge, decide how far to urge a specific treatment, and how far simply to comply with what the patient has heard from a neighbour is a good treatment. In other words, interpretation and insight are components of the judgements of the scientist and the clinician. But the good doctor must, in addition, be sensitive to the ethical nature of the doctor–patient relationship. The ethics of that relationship involves not only the use of principles of ethics, but also the exercise of virtues, such as compassion, equanimity, and courage. Interpretation, insight, and ethical sensitivity are expressed in humane judgement. There is a second main component of humane judgement: educatedness. The good doctor is not only trained but broadly educated, where that involves being adaptable, being developed as a rounded person, and having a broad perspective. 'Humane judgement', understood as ethically sensitive and educated judgement, is the other main component of good clinical judgement.

It must be remembered that there is a domain in medicine other than the clinical, namely the public. The scientific evidence-base of public health medicine derives from epidemiology, which might seem an objective, neutral, judgement-free science, but judgement is involved in several ways. First, and most obviously, it is involved in deciding what to do with the findings as a matter of public policy. For example, should there be a 'girls only' policy with respect to the rubella vaccine or a 'girls and boys' policy? The answer to this question involves an amalgam of the technical and the moral/political. Second, and less obviously, the decision about which epidemiological studies to undertake in the first place involves the same judgmental mixture of the technical and the moral/political. Epidemiology, therefore, is not immune to judgement.

The questions of whether there is a need for health-care rationing, and if so, how it should be implemented, are important in every industrialized country. We believe that the evidence points clearly to this need. But the designing and implementation of systems of rationing involve moral and political judgements at both the macro and the micro levels. Judgements in this sphere are highly controversial.

The final chapter of the book was concerned with how, if at all, the medical curriculum can be widened to aid the development of the humane attitude, or how medical training can become truly medical education. We suggested that Special Study Modules could help here, with the blessing of the GMC. It may be that tutors in postgraduate medical education could try something similar. In an Appendix we have provided an account of two such SSMs, one of which, in philosophy, has already been piloted at Glasgow through the co-operation of the Departments of Philosophy and General Practice. It is through this kind of co-operation, in a University setting, that the broad educational aspects of the medical curriculum can be realized. This will result in the creation of 'the good doctor', the clinician whose technical judgements are fully integrated with humane judgements.

Appendix to Chapter 6:
Some Possible Courses

Having described the way in which the SSM can contribute to introducing arts and humanities subjects to medical curricula, we will now outline two courses which have been designed for medical students taking SSMs. One is in literature and the other in philosophy. The philosophy module has already been taken by two intakes of 10 second year medical students and we shall describe their response to it, including how they felt it contributed to their development as doctors. By describing the two courses we hope to demonstrate that students will experience a broadening of their educational experience practically—as they will be taught by non-medical teachers and along with arts students—and also that it is a different kind of experience. As we have just discussed in 6.8, an objectives-led approach to education which focuses on the *outcome* of the education is not appropriate for courses which aim to develop students' awareness of their personal attributes so the courses focus on a *process*-based approach.

1. An SSM on Literature

We will describe this module in terms of literature but it would be adaptable, if resources were available, to other arts or some mixture of arts.

For this module to be successful it is important that we attract the right number of enthusiastic students to take it. They are likely to be offered a wide selection of SSMs. How are they to appreciate what this course will have to offer? Many students are attracted to the new curricula being offered by medical schools and appreciate the change in emphasis from training to education. This SSM expresses the new medical education ethos and will interest students because it will enable them to explore aspects of medical practice in a novel way. Moreover, increased personal contact between students and their teachers in the new curricula also facilitates the dissemination of new ideas in medical education. This module provides a unique opportunity for personal contact and fruitful discussion between students and staff on a wide range of topics pertinent to medical education. It should be noted that courses like this have been run in the past on a voluntary basis both in Glasgow[1] and Melbourne[2] to the acclaim of students.

(a) The course

We propose a four week course which will involve the participation of:

- Students in small groups
- University-based tutors from different departments and faculties
- 'Expert' lecturers to participate in the plenary week.

There will be an introductory week, which will include staff and students from all participating departments. The week will be built around a single theme : 'The Links Between Literature and Medicine'. Activities will be mainly small group based and will include:

- Expert presentations and workshops e.g. creative writing, literary criticism, philosophy of literature, other art forms.
- Discussing in small tutor led groups a prescribed set of literary works which have been read in advance.
- Discussion of a piece of work selected in advance by each student for its relevance to the theme of the week.
- A group project of a literary nature to be presented at the end of the week. The scope for this is wide but might include the performance of a short play, the designing of a magazine, or some form of creative writing.
- Discussions between individuals and tutors aiming at identifying projects to be worked on for the rest of the module.

- 'Field visits'—evening attendances at theatres, poetry readings etc.

For the rest of the module the students of each group will work on the assignments they have chosen individually under the guidance of their tutor. Most of this time will be spent in private study but there will be at least 2 tutorial sessions per week, one for the group to meet together and another for the tutor to meet each student separately to discuss their work. The groups will meet again at the end of the module for one day for the reading of creative work and for an evaluation of the module to be carried out.

(b) Assessment

The students' assessment will be based on 2 assignments which they will decide on during the course of the plenary week and work on for the rest of the module.

1. Submitted Essay (minimum 2000 words).

This should be related in some way to medicine and should show evidence of appropriate reading and a critical approach to its analysis.

Suitable titles might be;

(a) Take any one or more novels of the nineteenth century in which death and dying play a prominent role. Analyse the attitudes expressed and compare them with our own.

(b) Discuss the portrayal of the doctor in the plays of Ibsen. How can doctors learn from a study of these works?

(c) What can be learned from Wordsworth's poem 'The Idiot Boy' about human attitudes to mental handicap?

(d) Discuss the evolution of the medical soap opera.

2. Creative Piece/Literary Criticism

The second assignment would involve students in some creative writing or (if they do not feel able to do this) an in-depth literary criticism of a work which they would choose with the guidance of their tutor. The main specification should be a relevance to medicine, though a broad view of this relationship is important.

(c) Conclusion

We have outlined an SSM in Medicine and Literature. The impetus towards designing this course has come from the GMC who are expecting medical schools to include a wide range of subjects—not just medical—within the new framework. Literature seems to fit closely the GMC requirements for the content of an SSM. Equally important, it offers an alternative educational approach which stresses the 'process' rather than the 'outcome' of the course. Thus, the course certainly aims to develop an understanding of the main themes by means of personal inquiry, and the structure of the course encourages this as it is consists of a mixture of individual reading followed, and supported by, reflective and interactive small groups. Furthermore, by having the aim of understanding as the only predicted outcome, this development can proceed in many different directions, all of which may be appropriate, without the fear that the students are 'not doing what they're supposed to'. This model allows greater freedom for the teaching of the course while maximising the learning. It is neither appropriate nor desirable that the outcome of the module (expressed in performance objectives) should dictate and even stultify the achievements of the students involved. It is, therefore, an appropriate module for developing the humane attitude which some influential doctors have found lacking in contemporary medicine[3]. As Sir William Osler put it: 'the humanities are the hormones',[4] they catalyse thought and humanize practice.

2. An SSM on Philosophy: The Individual in Society

In February 1998 the first student intake into the new medical curriculum at Glasgow University took their first group of SSMs and ten of them chose to do a module in philosophy. The title of the module was, 'The Individual in Society; an introduction to social and political philosophy'. This module was a collaboration between the departments of general practice and philosophy and this enabled the medical students to take part of a course which was being taught to students of philosophy in their first year. There are problems with laying on arts courses in medicine and the main one is getting teachers who are prepared to take on the extra burden of teaching medical students. The model provided by this collaboration, where the module 'piggy-backed' on a course in philosophy, may be a useful one for other courses.

It seemed particularly appropriate to include philosophy amongst the first group of SSM options that students could take at Glasgow. The GMC in *Tomorrow's Doctors* said that:

'The modules offered will depend on the interests, resources and individual enthusiasms of medical school staff and to some extent on the wider range of opportunities within their universities.' (p.9)

Glasgow University has a long standing tradition in philosophy and major figures such as Francis Hutcheson, Adam Smith and Thomas Reid were at one time professors of philosophy there. Philosophy has long been considered a central subject in the MA degree. Centuries of endorsement of the educational value of the study of philosophy would certainly be an encouragement to those of us who are interested in education but the course needs to be justified in terms of its relevance to the future development of medical students as doctors.

We will describe the course—it aims, structure and assessment—and go on to show how the two main aims are related to the education of doctors. The question of whether the course succeeded in its long term purpose of broadening the outlook of future doctors cannot yet be answered, but we will describe the initial evaluation by the students and their assessment of whether the course was valuable for them.

(a) The course

The course had two main aims:

1) To encourage the students to adopt the techniques of philosophical analysis in their approach to an argument; and

2) To expose them to the broadening experience of an academic culture different from their own.

The first aim relates to the fact that philosophy can teach students to think and argue in a valid and coherent way. The second aim refers to the idea of a counter culture which we have already discussed (6.5) and relates more to the actual experience of doing the module rather than its content. We will say more about these aims and their importance in the context of medical education later.

The module provided ten second year medical students with the opportunity to spend five weeks studying Plato's *Republic* in the context of a course of lectures on political philosophy. SSMs have the advantage that they are 5 weeks blocks set aside from the rest of the course and students can concentrate solely on their module subjects during this time. The medical students were, therefore, able to fit in with a pre-existing course on political philosophy which was about to start at the same time as their module. The lectures and reading material from this course became part of the module. The co-existence of the two courses had another advantage in that the medical students were taught alongside the arts faculty students and were taught by philosophers who were not specially angling their material at a medical audience. These points are important in terms of the second aim, that of exposing the students to a different academic culture.

The lectures were delivered by two lecturers, one dealing with the text of *The Republic* in some detail, and the other giving an overview of political philosophy from Hobbes onwards. Two seminars involving the whole group were held each week on Mondays and Fridays. The Monday seminar focused on the understanding and analysis of argument. The students were set an analytical exercise to do at the start of the module and one at the end to see how their analytical skills had progressed. The Friday seminar clarified points raised in relation to the lectures and the reading of the set text. Two seminar papers were set to guide and focus the students' reading, one on 'Plato's views on education', and the other, 'Plato's view of the family'. Apart from attending these classes the students spent their time reading, writing and, most importantly, thinking.

Assessment of the module consisted of three parts:

1) The class essay, consisting of 70% of the marks. Students were given a choice of two titles: 'Do we have a moral obligation to obey the laws of the state?' and, 'To what extent can one justify the criticisms of democracy which Plato's makes in *The Republic* ?';

2) Two seminar papers, contributing a total of 20%; and

3) The second analytical exercise, which gained 10%.

The students were, therefore, kept quite busy during the module, being involved in an educational experience quite different from what they had encountered at university so far. Most of them had not studied philosophy before and they had certainly not experienced the kind of teaching structure that the module provided. The content of the module, in that they were studying Plato and more general political philosophy, was entirely new to all of them. These issues raise the question of justification of the module in the context of medical education. Of what benefit is five weeks of philosophy to medical students, and why should they learn about Plato? In answering these two questions we shall return to a consideration and justification of the two aims of the module.

(b) Why philosophy for medical students?

We have already discussed the subject of transferable skills (6.7.2) and this module is an example of a non-medical subject which can teach doctors in training useful skills. One of the major criticisms levelled at recent medical education has been that students, particularly in the pre-clinical years of their education, have been so busy digesting large amounts of information, they have never had the opportunity to think for themselves. Once they start their clinical training, however, they are expected to be able to piece together the various bits of information that make up a case history and come to a logical conclusion on diagnosis. The main reason why philosophy has been a major part of university arts courses for hundreds of years is because it can teach people to think. Clinical diagnosis requires the doctors to be able to sort out information about a patient, order it and construct arguments for or against certain conclusions (diagnoses). Philosophy can teach students how to go about this, but also when conclusions can be strongly or weakly argued, or valid or invalid. A major part of the module focused on leaning about argument and students were taught the steps to take in constructing arguments.

Besides leaning how to do this for themselves, the students also learned to recognize when others were making arguments and when these arguments might be valid or invalid. This was a particular revelation to them (as we will show in the evaluation) as they had been used to accepting much of what they were told. Most of the students commented that they had begun to question received wisdom with much more confidence by the end of the module. In other words, they were beginning to adopt Enlightenment attitudes: *Sapere audi* or, in Kant's paraphrase, 'Have courage to use your own reason'[5].

These two skills, the ability to make an argument and the ability to identify and criticize the arguments of others, both relate to the first aim of the module. As skills, they were part of the training that the module provided. But learning about philosophy is also an educational activity (6.2) and part of the module's value here was that it distanced the students from the pervading culture of their medical education and medical class and placed them in the arts faculty (physically and intellectually) and amongst philosophy students and teachers. This was the second aim of the module: to provide a broadening academic experience and one that the students would recognize and value as different.

(c) Why should medical students study Plato's Republic?

The Republic was chosen as the set text for the module for reasons that are relevant to both of the module aims. To broaden their educational experience, the students read the text with a view to discussing and developing a view on the moral, cultural and political themes that were raised, many of which were as relevant in Plato's Athens as they are to us today. In relation to learning about argument, *The Republic* presents a series of arguments that the students could discuss and analyse.

There are a number of parallels between the society of Athens and our own. Athens was a democracy much influenced by public speakers and this mirrors our society where the media have a similarly powerful role. Greece was a collection of city states, a bit like modern Europe, with some in Greece wanting unification. The issue of European union is a hot one in this country at the moment, particularly in relation to currency union. Education is a central issue in *The Republic* and is one that closely concerned the students who were taking the module as they were the first group to experience the new style of medical education at the University and their views and reactions are being constantly sought. The students were asked to write seminar papers on Plato's discussion of education and on his view of the family.

The study of *The Republic* was set in the context of a series of lectures on social and political philosophy and one of the 'core' themes emphasized by the GMC in *Tomorrow's Doctors* (p.17) is 'Man and Society'. By this the GMC were thinking mainly of human development and sociology and psychology relevant to medicine, as well as ethics. However, by studying *The Republic,* (and hearing about other themes in political philosophy in the lecture course) the medical students were able to consider some of the fundamental reasons why society exists in the first place. Plato deals with the reasons why people live together in communities : humans are frail beings and need the protection of a group, and there is a need to share human resources in the form of the diverse range of talents that people have. Without reference to religious morality, Plato deals with the moral values which, of necessity, must rule human society granted these human needs and vulnerabilities. This approach opened the students minds to a deeper understanding of the origins of our society's make up and of the values which allow it to function.

These issues are all part of our modern social and political agenda and it is important for any educated member of our society to have a view on them. In *The Republic* these issues are raised for the students' consideration in a controversial way as the book takes the form of a series of dialogues between Socrates and the various young men of Athens. This structure encouraged the students to form their own views, as they found themselves agreeing or disagreeing with the protagonists in the dialogue, and enhanced their understanding of the construction of arguments.

We hoped, therefore, that both the content as well as the structure of the teaching of the module would help the students to develop the ability to express their views coherently, constructively and, most of all, with convincing arguments.

(d) Evaluation of the module

Having discussed what happened in the module and what its ambitious aims were, it is important to give an idea of whether the module achieved these aims or not: did we manage to turn the students into philosophers? Evaluation was carried out in two ways, firstly, by a conventional questionnaire, which asked the students about their reasons for taking the module and what they thought of the structure, content and educational value of the module; and secondly, by comparing the two analytical exercises that the students did at the beginning and end of the module, to see how their analytical skills had progressed.

Turning first to the results of the questionnaire. Most of the students had taken the module because they were keen to do an arts subject again, having missed the opportunity to study the arts since leaving school and nine out of the ten wanted a complete change from medicine. We asked the students' views on the fact that we did not set knowledge objectives for the course in the form of a learning contract and they were all in favour of this. They did feel, however, that they required more feedback on how they were doing. The students felt stimulated by the discussion in seminars and by the new ideas that were introduced. They were keen for more discussion time and more time spent on clarifying issues they did not understand from their reading and lectures. The group seemed to have handled the content of the module well and most felt subjectively that they were better able to analyse argument by the end of the course. Most also said that they would be able to describe the major arguments of *The Republic* to a friend.

Turning to the students' views of the educational value of the module for themselves, all had discussed the module with their colleagues indicating that we had achieved an important prerequisite for an educational process—that the students had become interested and engaged in what they were doing (c.f. 6.2). Most of them, indeed, wanted to do more philosophy in the future and had ideas they wished to pursue. They were asked specifically about the value of the module in medical educational terms and the most frequent comment here was that they would now be less inclined to accept things that they were told without justification and that they would be more critical of what they were told.

The second part of the evaluation involved a comparison of the first and second analytical exercises as a more objective measure of whether the students had succeeded in learning the skills of analysis. All of the students displayed some improvement, in terms both of the organisation and content of their analysis, over the course of the module.

In summary, then, this module was designed to broaden both the students' education and their views of society and its structures and the process by which it helped them to do this enabled them to learn the techniques of philosophical argument and how to apply it themselves. The initial evaluation would imply that we has succeeded in the short term. A concluding comment made by one of the group about the module was that

'It has opened my mind'.

We hope that they will continue into the rest of their education as doctors with open minds.

References

1. Calman KC, Downie RS, Duthie M, Sweeney B, Literature and medicine: a short course for medical students. *Medical Education* 1988; 22: 265–69.
2. Moore AR, Medical humanities—a new medical adventure. *New England Journal of Medicine* 1976; 293: 1479–80.
3. Weatherall DJ, The inhumanity of medicine. *BMJ* 1994; 309: 1671–2.
4. Osler W. *The Old Humanities and the New Science.* Boston: Houghton Mifflin, 1920. p. 26
5. Broadie A (ed.) *The Scottish Enlightenment: An Anthology.* Edinburgh: Canongate Classics 1997, p.1.

Index